Essential Practice for Healthcare Assistants

Essential Practice for Healthcare Assistants

Edited by
Angela Grainger

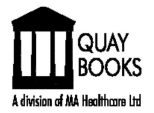

QUAY
BOOKS

A division of MA Healthcare Ltd

Quay Books Division, MA Healthcare Ltd, St Jude's Church, Dulwich Road, London
SE24 0PB

British Library Cataloguing-in-Publication Data
A catalogue record is available for this book

Printed by CLE, Huntingdon, Cambridgeshire

CONTENTS

CONTRIBUTORS

Lesley Baillie RGN, RNT, BA(Hons), MSc, PhD. Principal Lecturer, Faculty of Health and Social Care, South Bank University, London

Angela Grainger RGN, RSCN, RCNT, PG. Dip. Nursing (Lond), Further Ed. Teacher's Cert, MA, PhD. Assistant Director of Nursing, King's College Hospital NHS Foundation Trust, London.

Ann Pegram RGN, BSc, Post Grad. Cert. Education, M. Phil. Lecturer, Florence Nightingale School of Nursing & Midwifery, King's College, London.

Vinice Thomas RGN, BSc(Hons), MBA, PGDip (Education). Assistant Director of Nursing/Clinical Governance, Acting Director of Infection and Prevention and Control, Harrow Primary Care Trust, and currently on secondment to the Department of Health, Healthcare Associated Infection and Cleanliness Division as part of the National Improvement Team.

Sarah Mackie RGN, BSc, Post. Grad. Dip. Critical Care. Practice Development Nurse, Renal Care Division, King's College Hospital NHS Foundation Trust.

Menna Lloyd-Jones RGN, SCM, MSc, Dip N, PGCE. Senior Nurse Tissue Viability, Wales.

Sue Foxley RGN, MSc. Consultant Nurse, Continence Care, King's College Hospital NHS Foundation Trust.

Carol Haigh RGN, PhD. Professor of Nursing, Manchester Metropolitan University.

Catherine Bryant FRCP. Consultant Physician, Department of Gerontology, King's College Hospital NHS Foundation Trust.

Emma Ouldred RGN, BSc, MSc. Dementia Clinical Nurse Specialist, Department of Gerontology, King's College Hospital NHS Foundation Trust.

Chris Barber RGN, BSc(Hons), M.Ed. Agency Nurse (learning disability).

ACKNOWLEDGEMENTS

I wish to thank all of the chapter authors for their contributions and supportive enthusiasm. I also wish to thank Maria Anguita, Associate Publisher at Quay Books, for her unwavering support in getting the book to press.

Most of all I wish to thank you, our readers, because without you this book would never have come into being. I hope you all have very happy careers in health care.

FOREWORD

Healthcare delivery in the 21st century depends increasingly on multiprofessional teamwork. This means that each member of the team understands and works within the scope of their practice, carrying on to deliver optimal care to patients that is timely, appropriate, and where possible evidence-based.

Healthcare assistants are a valuable and increasingly important part of the wider team of healthcare professionals.

The contributors to this book have direct and up-to-date experience in the recruitment, training, management and professional development of healthcare assistants and of working alongside them.

Many healthcare assistants, whether new or experienced, feel the need for an uncluttered textbook of key principles of clinical practice, skills and policy which has been developed specifically with healthcare assistants in mind. This book has been produced with the intent of fulfilling at least a substantial part of this need.

I hope this book also does something else that is important, which is to demonstrate to all healthcare assistants who use it regularly, or to those who merely browse though it, that members of the multidisciplinary team respect and value the work that healthcare assistants do, and seek to welcome, encourage and guide you in the practice of this essential and rewarding career.

Dame Jacqueline Docherty DBE
Chief Executive, West Middlesex University Hospital NHS Trust,
Formerly Deputy Chief Executive and Director of Nursing and Operations,
King's College Hospital NHS Foundation Trust, London

INTRODUCTION

Providing holistic, person-centred care is the goal of every healthcare professional. Healthcare assistants are part of the nursing family and as such share in the giving of direct, and on occasions, intimate, care. You may be providing care to the patient or the service user, or to their close family and friends.

How patients and service users experience the receipt of care is very important. Considerate and competent care enhances trust and confidence in the service and in those who provide it, whilst poor or inadequate care can lead to service users disengaging from the service, and also to complaints. Those who are very ill, frail, or dependent might easily feel completely at the mercy or whim of those attending them, and even one bad experience can make such a patient or service-recipient very wary of what might be coming next. Establishing a good rapport with patients and their families, and being confident that your professional knowledge and skill is contributing to the delivery of high-quality competent care will enhance your feeling of work being done well and that you have chosen the right vocation.

This book has two aims. First, to explain the theory that underpins the fundamental basics of care-giving which are part of the core duties of most healthcare assistants, regardless of the care setting or environment. Second, to increase the healthcare assistant's job satisfaction by showing how the fundamental basics of care delivery fit into the wider framework of holistic yet individualised care.

These aims dovetail into the learning principles and learning techniques discussed in the book's final chapter on work-based learning. On this point, it is hoped that this book will stimulate those readers who are interested in the possibility of progressing to become a registered healthcare practitioner, whether in nursing, midwifery, or the allied health professions such as physiotherapy, occupational therapy, speech and language therapy, dietetics, podiatry, or chiropody, to consider undertaking the required vocational education and training.

This is a generalist textbook, and as such it covers most aspects of generic (applicable to all) practice. Fundamental practice is demonstrated in the chapters on maintaining privacy and dignity, infection control, understanding the skin in relation to personal hygiene, pressure ulcer prevention, and principles of wound healing and management, nutrition, elimination needs and catheter care, clinical observations, and communication and documentation.

The chapter on work-based learning will help you to maximise the learning opportunities that come your way by virtue of having direct contact with patients facing all sorts of situations. This will help improve and advance your knowledge, understanding, skills, and competence, which, in turn, ensures that the patient has a better experience, time after time.

Certain other subjects covered are more specialised and include managing pain and providing comfort, caring for sick children, common mental health problems in older adults, caring for the person who has learning disabilities, and spirituality. This is because holistic care takes account of the need to meet not only a patient's generic requirements, but any additional issues facing the patient, and/or the patient's family. These can be either physical or emotional needs, or a combination of the two. Moreover some patient and service-user groups have a distinctive need to have even generic aspects of care modified and adapted to take account of their unique perspective of their situations. This includes children, older people, and those who have a learning disability or an intellectual impairment. The chapters focusing on the principles of care-giving for these patients will show you how you can apply an understanding of these principles so that you can approach the patient appropriately, explain the need for certain procedures in a way the patient can understand and accept, and perform the required act of care with no, or minimal, upset to the patient.

The chapters in this book can be read as stand-alone chapters, or the book can be read in sequence. Each chapter is referenced. Some of the chapters include information on practical care aspects discussed in other chapters. This is to emphasise that some fundamental aspects of care have an associated additional meaning, depending on the context of care. Examples include oral hygiene (mouth care) as part of fundamental personal hygiene. Malnourished or immune-suppressed patients might require additional oral care and certain special mouthwashes might be prescribed. This is therefore also discussed in the chapter on nutrition.

All learning should be interesting and fun, otherwise we are less likely to be motivated to learn. You might find, for example, that although you have minimal personal contact with children or with people who have a learning disability, reading the chapters focusing on their care needs whets your appetite for finding out more and perhaps to think about working especially with them.

Whilst much of the content of this book is generic, all of the contributing authors share a belief that all practice, whatever its nature and irrespective of the care setting, is special. This is because individual patients are at the centre of care-giving practices, and in fact patients are the sole reason for us engaging in any care-planning activities in the first place. It is a sobering thought that we receive our salaries or wages because a patient or a service user is ill, or is otherwise dependent on us to meet his/her needs. It is the relationship with our patients and service users that make each episode of care-giving unique, and therefore special.

Even if patients or their relatives are difficult to please and we struggle to get things 'right', there is a learning opportunity here in trying to see things from the other person's perspective. This in turn helps us to acquire deeper understanding of the issues which people face when they are in our care, and helps us to develop empathy regarding how their situation seems to them, rather than only how it seems to us. Through reflective practice we can consider how we might improve things by responding differently next time we face a similar situation. This should result in a constant improvement in professional relationships and standards of care, and should reduce the likelihood of care-giving being fraught or stressful for the patient, relative, or for the healthcare professional. It can be helpful to realise that at the end of a particularly busy shift we as professional staff get to go home, whereas, for the time being at least, our patients may not be able to. On top of this, some of our patients may be encumbered by their physical body no longer working for them in the way that it used to, or they may be depressed by their health issues or by their physical limitation within an environment which is 'not theirs' and is not under their control. Remember, too, that when we go home, our patients do not cease to exist until we return therefore, unlike the healthcare professionals, they do not experience their health problems in manageable shifts but continuously.

Please do use this book as a resource tool. Also ask questions of what you read and discuss either the content, or the issues raised in the book, with your registered nurse clinical supervisor. Also read relevant professional healthcare journals, and attend in-house study days, as all of these activities feed the inquiring mind and as a result you learn more and feel more satisfied in what you do, and how you do it.

Angela Grainger

CHAPTER I

Maintaining privacy and dignity

Lesley Baillie

Whether or not people's privacy and dignity needs are maintained affects their perceptions of their whole healthcare experience. Therefore preserving privacy and dignity is central in all care activities you carry out with patients and clients. This chapter addresses the following areas:

● The meaning of privacy and dignity
● A background to privacy and dignity in care
● Loss of privacy and dignity in care
● Maintaining privacy and dignity in care
● Dealing with situations where privacy and dignity are threatened.

For simplicity, the terms patient/client are used throughout this chapter to refer to people you are caring for. However, healthcare assistants work with a wide range of people in different settings and you might more appropriately refer to the people who you care for as residents or service users, or you might work with children, young people and families.

The meaning of privacy and dignity

Privacy and dignity are often spoken about together but it is useful to distinguish between them while considering how they are linked. First think for a few moments about the terms 'privacy' and 'dignity' and try writing down what you think they mean. Now think about what privacy and dignity might mean to patients and clients in your particular care setting. You might have found it easiest to define privacy. There are different aspects of privacy and all of these can be affected during healthcare.

Privacy of space
Most people have some private space of their own, but in health care private

space may be minimal and can be easily breached. In hospitals patients have very little private space at all. In the community, patients' homes are entered by healthcare workers and their home space can become full of healthcare equipment, encroaching on personal space.

Privacy of the body

This aspect of privacy relates to modesty, which is a requirement in some religions and also has cultural influences. There are societal 'norms' about bodily exposure — how much of the body is exposed, in front of whom, and in what situation. For example, a woman may feel perfectly at ease undressing in front of strangers in a single sex changing room at the gym but may feel acutely embarrassed about being dressed in a gown in a mixed sex bay in hospital. People often have to expose their bodies to healthcare workers during their treatment and care. In some religions, bodily exposure to people of the opposite sex causes considerable distress. Patients' feelings about bodily exposure can also be influenced by their age, upbringing and body image.

Privacy of information

Confidentiality in health care must be maintained but there are many opportunities for information about patients (written, verbal or electronic) to be seen or heard by other people. Communicating information about patients between healthcare workers is necessary for safe treatment and care but information should not be shared unnecessarily. Patients or visitors should not overhear or see confidential information. This can be difficult to prevent in some settings, for example, multi-patient bays with minimal space between beds. Community patients usually keep their own case notes which could potentially be read by families or neighbours.

The meaning of dignity can be difficult to explain and people often have different interpretations of its meaning. However, as the Social Care Institute for Excellence (SCIE) (2006) has said:

> *'While dignity may be difficult to define, what is clear is that people know when they have not been treated with dignity and respect.'*
>
> *SCIE (2006)*

Dignity

SCIE (2006) suggests that dignity includes overlapping aspects such as respect, privacy, autonomy and self-worth. Therefore, you might think of privacy as being an aspect of dignity, but dignity is more than just privacy. A patient could feel that their privacy has been protected yet still feel that they have lost their dignity. However, if privacy is breached, it is unlikely that someone will feel that their dignity was preserved as they may feel that they were treated with a lack of respect or as if they are of no value.

Dignity relates to how people feel about themselves (e.g. self-worth), how they behave and how others behave towards them (e.g. being respectful). The Royal College of Nursing's (RCN) (2008a) definition of dignity (see *Box 1.1*) includes all these aspects and also highlights how people feel when their dignity is present (e.g. in control) and how people feel when dignity is absent (e.g. humiliated). The RCN (2008a) identifies that dignity is affected by the physical care environment and also by organisational culture, which includes aspects such as managerial support for dignity in care. The definition refers to people who have a lack of capacity which could relate to some patients you work with, for example if they have advanced dementia or are unconscious following a stroke. But as the RCN's (2008a) definition makes clear, dignity applies to everyone.

People who lack capacity are some of our most vulnerable patients and clients and we must be absolutely vigilant that their dignity is maintained.

Box 1.1 *Dignity*, a definition

Dignity is concerned with how people feel, think and behave in relation to the worth or value of themselves and others. To treat someone with dignity is to treat them as being of worth, in a way that is respectful of them as valued individuals.

In care situations, dignity may be promoted or diminished by: the physical environment; organisational culture; by the attitudes and behaviour of nurses and others and by the way in which care activities are carried out.

When dignity is present people feel in control, valued, confident, comfortable and able to make decisions for themselves. When dignity is absent people feel devalued, lacking control and comfort. They may lack confidence and be unable to make decisions for themselves. They may feel humiliated, embarrassed or ashamed.

Dignity applies equally to those who have capacity and to those who lack it. Everyone has equal worth as human beings and must be treated as if they are able to feel, think and behave in relation to their own worth or value.

Nurses should, therefore, treat all people in all settings and of any health status with dignity, and dignified care should continue after death.

Source: RCN (2008a)

The RCN also refers to treating people with dignity after death. Although it can be assumed that a person will not be aware of how they are treated after their death, it is of utmost importance to families that their deceased relatives' care is carried out with dignity, for example, that religious preferences are respected, privacy is maintained, the body is well presented and personal belongings are handled with care.

Dignity and privacy are linked concepts and they underpin all care activities. The next section provides a background to privacy and dignity in care and gives an overview of relevant legislation, professional issues and health policies and also outlines recent campaigns on privacy and dignity issues.

A background to privacy and dignity in care

Both legislation and health policies refer to privacy and dignity. The background to modern day human rights legislation is that in 1948 the United Nations (established in 1945 at the end of the Second World War) published 'The Universal Declaration of Human Rights' (UDHR), which recognized the 'inherent dignity' of human beings. 'Inherent dignity' refers to the belief that all human beings have dignity because they are humans. The UDHR included the statement:

> *'All human beings are born free and equal in dignity and rights'.*
>
> *UDHR (1948, Article 1)*

The UDHR was incorporated into UK law when the Human Rights Act (1998) was passed. The Human Rights Act recognises that all individuals have minimal and fundamental human rights and two of the articles relate to dignity and privacy. Article 3 'Prohibition of torture' states that:

> *'No one should be subjected to torture or to inhuman or degrading treatment or punishment'.*
>
> *Human Rights Act (1998, Article 3)*

Given the nature of healthcare investigations and treatment, some patients might view their experience as inhuman or degrading. Article 8 'Right to respect for private and family life' states that:

> *'Everyone has the right to respect for his private and family life, his home and his correspondence'.*
>
> *Human Rights Act (1998, Article 8)*

As discussed in the previous section, threats to confidentiality and mixed sex accommodation are examples where patients may feel that their privacy is threatened.

Dignity is central to professional healthcare practice for nurses, doctors and allied health professionals, as is being incorporated into their professions' codes of conduct and ethics. As healthcare assistants work within professional healthcare teams, the same commitment to dignity and privacy is expected by patients and relatives, and is normally a requirement of employers.

Since the 1990s there has been media concern about the dignity of patients, particularly in acute care settings, but other areas too such as residential care. In 1997, a journalist, Martin Bright, reported in the *Observer* on the indignities experienced by his grandmother following a stroke. Following this article a Help the Aged-backed *Dignity on the Ward* campaign was launched, which initiated a Department of Health (DH) funded inquiry into the care of older people in acute hospitals in England. The inquiry report entitled *Not Because we Are Old* (Health Advisory Service [HAS], 2000) indicated that preserving dignity and individuality, when meeting essential needs, was not always achieved and although this sometimes related to a poor physical environment it was more often to do with staff attitudes. There was inadequate provision of essential personal care, and staff interactions which threatened dignity were evident. The report also found, however, that some wards, however, had a culture of respect for patients. In England, the report provided the trigger for health policies such as *Essence of Care* (DH, 2001a) and the *National Service Framework for Older People* (DH, 2001b). Since then, health and social care policy documents in all four UK countries have increasingly stressed the importance of dignity in care.

The DH (2006a) launched a *Dignity* campaign including a 10-point challenge (see *Box 1.2*), which refers to expectations of staff behaviour and attention to privacy. Read through the challenge in *Box 1.2* and consider these 10 points in relation to your care setting: how might you achieve these goals for the people you care for? For example, what choices can you offer in care? How can you help people to express their needs? Other organisations have also run campaigns about dignity and privacy:

- The Help the Aged *Dignity on the Ward* campaign is ongoing (see www. helptheaged.org.uk). Help the Aged's (2007) report *The Challenge of Dignity in Care: Upholding the rights of the individual* details principles underlying dignity in care and aspects of care which are important for dignity. The aspects identified are: communication, privacy, self-determination and autonomy, food and nutrition, pain and symptom control, personal hygiene, personal care and help at home, death with dignity, social inclusion. Help the Aged have produced a series of guides to assist hospital staff to promote dignified care, which relate to many of these areas

- In 2006, the British Geriatric Society (BGS) launched a campaign *Dignity Behind Closed Doors* (see www.bgs.org.uk) which aimed to raise awareness that '*people, whatever their age and physical ability, should be able to choose to use the toilet in private in all care settings*'. The BGS campaign resources include a leaflet clearly setting out what is good practice and what is poor practice when assisting people with using the toilet

- The RCN (2008b) launched the campaign *Dignity at the Heart of Everything We Do* (see www.rcn.org.uk) which includes a range of resources to help nurses, students and healthcare support workers promote dignity in care. The RCN has also lobbied the British government about care environment issues which affect privacy and dignity (e.g. mixed sex wards).

Box 1.2 The *Dignity* challenge

High quality services that respect people's dignity should:

1. Show zero tolerance towards all forms of abuse
2. Treat people with the same respect as you would want for yourself and your family
3. Treat each person as an individual
4. Ensure people are able to maintain maximum levels of independence, choice and control
5. Support people in expressing their needs
6. Respect people's rights to privacy
7. Ensure people can complain without fear of retribution
8. Work with patients' families and their partners in their care
9. Help people to maintain confidence and self-esteem
10. Alleviate people's loneliness and isolation.

Source: DH (2006a)

In your own care setting, find out about the effect of the health policies or campaigns discussed above. For example, is there auditing of privacy and dignity benchmarks, with action plans? Is there a local 'dignity champion'? What activities are going on to address dignity and privacy in care?

Loss of privacy in care

Various reports have identified deficits in dignified care for older people (Help the Aged, 2007; Healthcare Commission, 2007) and for people with learning disabilities (Mencap, 2007). However all people undergoing health and social care in any setting and of any age can be vulnerable to loss of dignity. Think about your own care setting: what might lead to loss of privacy and dignity for your patients or clients?

Lack of privacy, inadequate fundamental care, poor communication and attitudes, and a deficient care environment, are discussed next.

Lack of privacy

An earlier section identified three areas of privacy: personal space, the body and information. Breaches of privacy can occur in any of these areas — here are some examples:

- Patients may feel that their personal space has been breached when staff or others enter beyond closed curtains or a closed door without asking, or move patients' belongings around in their bedside lockers or other furniture without discussion
- Patients may feel that the privacy of their body is violated if they are unnecessarily exposed, for example, bedside curtains are not fully closed while they are undergoing personal care, their clothing is removed or disturbed without discussion or consent, or they are dressed in clothing that does not cover their body adequately
- Patients may experience a lack of confidentiality when others can overhear personal information, for example, about incontinence, their medical diagnosis or home circumstances.

Box 1.3 provides an example of a patient's experience of a breach of privacy in a hospital ward. The patient had a blocked catheter and was having a bladder washout performed when another ward staff member entered the curtains without warning to talk to the nurse. The patient could not clearly see who had entered the curtains and was acutely aware of his bodily exposure. As you will read in *Box 1.3*, not only was his privacy breached but the two staff members talked over him and ignored him. By entering the curtains without permission, the staff member breached the patient's personal space, saw his body exposed and also learned that he was having this procedure performed. The nurse carrying out the procedure, rather than asking the person to leave and covering the patient, instead engaged in conversation.

Inadequate fundamental care

There are many reports of poor fundamental care, for example, a Department of Health (2006b) survey identified lack of assistance with eating, hygiene

---

Box 1.3 A breach of privacy during a bladder washout

'A nurse comes in, draws the curtains round, so I'm there, I'm on my back, my frock's [nightshirt] up round my waist — my legs are apart — they've got a bowl in me and she's syringing me...she [another staff member] puts her head through the curtain. Chats to this nurse who's treating me. And I thought: *'What are you doing? as far as I know, you're not a nurse — you've not come in here for my benefit.'* I felt a bit annoyed and a bit embarrassed at the thought that someone who was not medical staff as far as I know [saw me exposed]. I don't know what they were talking about but it was nothing to do with me. So I got a bit narked [annoyed] and felt a bit embarrassed. And a certain loss of dignity because I was not in a very dignified position'. (Male patient in his 70s)

Source: Baillie (2007)

---

and elimination as threats to dignity. Woolhead et al (2005) identified a lack of attention to older people's appearance as threatening their dignity. In Hlén's (2004) study, patients reported that their dignity was violated by lack of fundamental care, for example not being assisted to wash following vomiting. Age Concern (2006) reported many instances of older people being left hungry in hospital. Patients experiencing inadequate fundamental care will feel uncomfortable, uncared for and unvalued as well as experiencing incontinence, hunger, thirst, pain and poor hygiene.

Poor communication and attitudes

Examples include healthcare workers being discourteous and disrespectful, not greeting patients politely, being curt or brusque with patients, not introducing themselves, talking over patients and ignoring them (as in *Box 1.4*). Help the Aged (2007) reported the common but unsatisfactory practice of talking to older people as though they are children and that the use of endearments such as 'sweetheart' or 'darling' are sometimes inappropriately used rather than the older person's preferred name. Rudeness, careless handling of patients' property and not respecting a person's culture and religious beliefs can all diminish dignity. Patients' dignity can be threatened when staff adopt an authoritarian attitude, for example 'telling' rather than 'asking' patients (Baillie, 2007). Unkindness, belittling or demeaning patients and not treating them as individuals all threaten dignity too. If staff fail to gain consent before carrying out procedures, do not offer choices, or provide explanations and involve patients in decisions, control is removed and independence is denied.

Deficient care environment

An RCN (2008a) survey identified that the physical environment and employing organisation have a major impact on whether nurses and other staff can promote dignity in care. A poor physical environment (unclean, insufficient toilets/bathrooms, lack of resources and equipment, mixed sex accommodation) hamper staff in their efforts to maintain privacy and dignity during healthcare. Employing organisations might not prioritise privacy and dignity and fail to provide the material and human resources necessary to support privacy and dignity in care.

Commonly reported dignity compromises

The Healthcare Commission (2007) reported on the dignity of older people in hospital and listed commonly received complaints about dignity compromises (see *Box 1.4*). Take a look at these examples and reflect on practice in your setting: do any of these occur often or occasionally? If so, why do you think these happen? You will see that many of these complaints arise from staff behaviour (e.g. form of address) but others concern the care environment (e.g. mixed sex accommodation).

Box 1.4 Common examples of compromises in dignity taken from complaints received by the Healthcare Commission

1 Being addressed in an inappropriate manner
2 Being spoken about as if they were not there
3 Not being given proper information
4 Not seeking their consent and/or not considering their wishes
5 Being left in soiled clothes
6 Being exposed in an embarrassing manner
7 Not being given appropriate food or help with eating and drinking
8 Being placed in mixed sex accommodation
9 Being left in pain
10 Being in a noisy environment at night causing lack of sleep
11 Having to use premises that are unclean and smelly (e.g. toilets, wards)
12 Lack of protection of personal property including personal aids (hearing or visual)
13 Being subjected to abuse and violent behaviour.

Source: Healthcare Commission (2007)

In practice, many patients and clients do have positive experiences of their privacy and dignity being maintained. It is 'everybody's business' to preserve privacy and dignity, and healthcare assistants who work directly with patients and clients have a very important role.

Maintaining privacy and dignity in care

During all your care activities with patients and clients, always aim to preserve their privacy, deliver a high standard of fundamental care, and communicate in a way which promotes dignity. The provision of high quality fundamental care (such as hygiene, continence and nutrition) is covered in other chapters in this book. A conducive care environment is also important for privacy and dignity, including: cleanliness, good décor, suitable and sufficient toilets and bathrooms, single sex accommodation, adequate space, functional equipment, sufficient and suitably trained staff, well-fitting curtains, and a supportive staff team who are committed to maintaining patients' dignity (RCN, 2008a).

There is always some potential for privacy and dignity to be compromised during care activities. Therefore always plan your actions carefully and consider how you will maintain privacy and use appropriate communication. Prepare carefully for the procedure, gather equipment, organise the environment, and ensure that any additional staff needed are available. Always consider how you might promote independence, even in a very small way, and how you can ensure that physical comfort is maintained.

Maintaining privacy

This section considers how you can maintain privacy of personal space, privacy of patients' bodies and confidentiality. Appropriate communication is paramount throughout when maintaining privacy.

Privacy of personal space

In this section we will consider how you can maintain privacy in people's own homes, when a patient or resident is in a single room, or when a patient is in a multi-bed area.

If you are working in people's own homes, your employers will have procedures which you should follow and these will include personal safety aspects. As regards privacy, if you can book appointments for your visits you will convey respect and provide patients with some control over their own environment. Knock on the door, and if this is your first visit or you are an infrequent visitor, introduce yourself and show your ID badge, also checking the identity of the person answering the door. Remind the person why you are there (e.g. '*As we discussed, I have come to change your wound dressing*'). Ask for permission to go in and only enter areas of the property that you need to for carrying out the activity, always checking with the patient first. For example: '*I'll need some water — can I get some from the kitchen?*', '*Can I get some clean pyjamas for you from your bedroom — where are they kept?*'

Be very careful about commenting on the person's property in a way that might be perceived as critical. You will however have to raise concerns about any safety issues (e.g. lack of heating, trip hazards) but you must be constructive and tactful, otherwise people can feel that their home and their privacy has been invaded. Some people living alone will not be able to answer the door because of their health condition and you will use a key to enter independently. However, still always knock first and as you open the door you can call out, for example: '*Hello, Mrs O'Brien, it's Sue, I'm just coming into the hall*'. Depending on the activity you are carrying out, and the room's position, and therefore potential for people to see in from the street, suggest pulling the curtains. Be aware of other people's presence, checking discreetly whether the patient actually wants their relative, friend or neighbour present during care for support or whether they would prefer to be alone with you.

When caring for people in single rooms in care homes or hospital, always knock before entering and ask if you can come in. Introduce yourself (if it is the first time of meeting or if the person may have forgotten you) and explain why you are there, checking that it is alright to continue: for example, '*I've come to check whether your catheter needs emptying, is that OK?*' The person will have limited furniture in which to keep their belongings — in hospital probably just a bedside locker and bed table, but they will have more furniture in a care home bedroom. Ask first before getting items out, for example: '*Is your wash bag in your locker, can I get it out for you?*' Close the door and cover any window on the door (with the shutters or curtain, as provided) when you are going to carry out care. Place an 'engaged' sign on the door as a deterrent to other staff to enter while care is being carried out. You can also tell colleagues that you are going to be in the room, assisting with hygiene for example, so they will be less likely to disturb you. If there is a curtain inside the door, pull this too for added privacy. When leaving the room, ensure that you have moved any furniture (e.g. bed table) back into the position the patient would like and that you have put back any items used. You can give back some control by asking where they would like items placed, for example: '*Where would you like me to put your hairbrush?*' Ensure the person can reach their call bell. If possible negotiate whether they would like the door left open or shut unless clinical needs dictate this (for example, an infection may require the door to be shut) always explain such situations. You can remind the person when you will be coming back next while also reassuring them that they can call if they need you earlier.

In multi-bed areas, patients have only bed curtains and often a small bedspace so they have potentially very little privacy at all. Whenever possible, assist patients to the toilet, bathroom or other private area for personal care. Ensure that you close doors and put an 'engaged' sign on the door. In toilets or bathrooms you may have a curtain inside which you can pull. Whenever possible, leave patients to use the toilet or shower or bath alone. However, risk assessment will indicate that some patients are unsafe to leave alone or might require your assistance for some or all aspects. Some patients are too unwell to leave the bedside or they may be confined to bed due to their medical condition. Explain to these patients that their curtains can be pulled whenever needed for privacy and if they cannot pull their curtains themselves reassure them that they can call you to do so. When pulling curtains, take care that the edges are pulled closely together. You should report ill-fitting curtains and ask that they are replaced. Many hospital settings have clips or notices which you can attach to the closed curtains warning 'do not enter'. When patients have curtains pulled round them, do not walk in without warning. If you need to enter the curtains before the patient calls you, ask first, for example: '*It's me, Chris, can I come in?*' As you enter curtains take care that you do not cause them to gap so others can see in. Show respect for people's belongings and furniture too. You may need to move their belongings to place healthcare equipment, but do ask first, for example: '*Can I move your book for a moment while I put this tray on the table?*' Ensure that you replace the items where the person would like them. People with visual impairments need to know exactly where they can find their belongings by touch.

Privacy of patients' bodies

Bodily privacy must be maintained as much as possible during care. There are many care activities during which patients and clients need to undress. As well as attention to environmental privacy, as discussed above, consider how you can minimise bodily exposure and how much undressing is really required. Sometimes traditions lead to bodily exposure, for example patients being expected to undress into nightclothes or hospital gowns long before it is necessary for staff convenience rather than patients' well-being. As well as causing bodily exposure, this practice also diminishes dignity, reducing individuality and leading to a power imbalance between staff who are dressed in uniforms or day clothes, and patients who are dressed in nightwear. Whenever possible assist patients to dress in their own clothes and if they have to wear nightclothes provide a dressing gown. When hospital gowns must be used for operations or examinations never expect a patient to walk around in one without a dressing gown. If there are no dressing gowns available, at the very least provide another hospital gown to wear like a dressing gown. There are newer versions of hospital gowns now available which are less exposing. Patients sitting out in a chair or wheelchair in nightwear or a gown must be covered up adequately, for example using a blanket to cover legs.

When patients need to undress for procedures or examinations, if they can undress unassisted leave them to do so unobserved and provide a gown and blanket to cover themselves after undressing. When you need to expose an area of the patient's body for a procedure, always ask first, for example, *'Can I lift up your nightdress?'* If possible ask the patient to move clothing themselves, and only move clothing the minimum amount necessary ensuring that the rest of the patient's body is covered. When washing a patient use towels and a sheet to cover areas of the body not being washed. Replace clothing as soon as possible.

When you need additional staff to help you during an exposing procedure (e.g. when assisting a patient onto the toilet who needs help from two people), always introduce them to the patient and explain why they are there. You may sometimes be asked to chaperone another staff member during an exposing procedure (e.g. a rectal examination), which is for protection of both the staff member and the patient. This increased 'audience' potentially causes further embarrassment for patients so always introduce yourself, giving your name and job role. Whenever possible, stand or sit where the patient can see you, talk to the person and avoid looking at their exposed body area.

Some patients do not wish to expose their bodies to staff of the opposite sex and certain religions may stipulate this requirement.

Maintaining confidentiality

Patients and clients are usually well aware that certain information about them must be shared between healthcare workers to ensure their safety, continuity of care and appropriate referrals. However, patients must be able to feel confident that information is not shared unnecessarily between healthcare workers, that it is not shared with their families or friends without their permission, and that their personal information is not shared with other patients, visitors or the media. Concerned families and friends will often request information about patients but always ask the patient concerned what information they would like you to pass onto the enquirer and if possible, enable them to talk to their relative or friend themselves. There will probably be policies about information-giving in your workplace — do ensure that you work within your employers' policies. When information is passed between team members (e.g. during a ward handover), the environment used should ensure that other people do not overhear.

Confidentiality is generally easier to achieve in patients' own homes but it is more challenging in hospitals particularly when working in multi-patient areas. Pulling curtains provides a visual barrier, but auditory privacy can still be breached. For this reason, taking patients to private areas is always preferable. If you have to carry out care at the bedside, you can be discreet in your communication. Ensure that patients with hearing impairments have working hearing aids in place and can see you when you are talking to them. Keep your voice low and use non-verbal communication to support your verbal communication. When communicating with other staff about care in a multi-bed area, consider who might overhear. For example, if you are dealing with incontinence, fetch other staff or equipment discreetly. Instances where a healthcare worker calls out for an incontinence pad for a patient loudly across a ward are not acceptable. Also consider how you can deal discreetly with any smells that might occur, ensuring that you do not refer to them verbally or non-verbally and use any strategies such as window-opening or sprays in a quiet and discreet manner.

Communication and attitudes to promote dignity

While privacy is crucial for maintaining dignity, communication and attitudes are also very important. In Baillie's (2007) research, a patient described the nurse who had cared for him and maintained his dignity as being:

> '...sensitive, explains what she's going to do before she does it, she's cheerful, she has a sense of humour, she appears interested in me as an individual, she has a caring approach, appears to enjoy her work - doesn't appear as though it's a chore'.
>
> *Baillie (2007)*

When you communicate with patients and clients consider how you can help them to feel comfortable, in control and valued.

Communication which helps people to feel comfortable

Patients will feel comfortable with healthcare workers who have a sensitive approach, display empathy and develop a relationship with them. Humour can help patients feel comfortable, and it is sometimes used by patients themselves as a way of relieving embarrassment. However staff using humour must do so sensitively and appropriately. Patients will feel comfortable when staff are friendly and reassuring to them. Professionalism from staff will help patients to feel safe in their hands and therefore comfortable in their care.

Communication which helps people to feel in control

A loss of control can cause a loss of dignity. Providing explanations and information can help patients to feel more in control of what is happening to them, and enable them to give informed consent. Where possible, offer choices to patients and enable their independence and involvement. Consider how verbal and written information can be presented in a way that people can understand. Interpreters can be used with patients who cannot speak English, but there are issues of privacy and confidentiality. For example, it is usually inappropriate to use a family member to interpret, although in an emergency there may be no immediate alternative. A professional interpreter who is from the same community as the patient may not be acceptable either. Interpreters, whether family or professional, should usually be of the same sex unless the patient requests otherwise. Written information should be available in languages which are spoken locally. As well as language issues, verbal and written information should be appropriate for the patient's age and level of understanding, with information suitable for people with learning disabilities. Pictures and photographs can be helpful for explaining information.

Communication which helps people to feel valued

Patients will feel valued if you listen to them and give them time, show concern for them as individuals, and are considerate and helpful towards them. Courteousness is very important so always be polite and respectful in your communication, for example greeting patients, introducing yourself and asking how they would like to be addressed. Ensure that you respect cultural and religious beliefs, providing any facilities necessary, for example, prayer.

Box 1.5 includes two examples from nurses of how privacy and dignity can be maintained for patients during care activities. As you can see, both examples include careful planning, preparing appropriate equipment, thoughtfulness, patient involvement, attention to privacy, and effective communication.

Dealing with situations where dignity and privacy are threatened

Many patients are vulnerable to their privacy and dignity being diminished in healthcare because of their health conditions and the associated care and treatment. Your own commitment to patients' privacy and dignity will have a very valuable impact on their healthcare experience. But you should also consider how you might respond if you see colleagues behaving in a way that compromises privacy and dignity or if the care environment provides a barrier.

Box 1.5 Maintaining privacy and dignity during care activities

Assisting a person with Parkinson's disease with eating
Modified diets are served onto everyday plates; use of the correctly sized spoon or fork; where there is dribbling, the use of a tissue to clean excess; the involvement of the individual in the activity (even in a small way); privacy is offered; verbal interactions with the individual are adult and not infantile; checking to see that the individual in comfortable with the way that I am 'assisting' them; the individual is offered the opportunity to wash their hands before and after the meal (even if they will play no part in the activity); care is taken to not spill food, but if clothes are soiled, assistance is given to change them. (Ward Manager, acute hospital)

Bed bath
Patient involved in discussion about care for the day and is in agreement. Ensure that I have all equipment I require. Ensure I have an assistant to facilitate safe moving and handling. Inform colleagues that I will be undertaking bed bath. Ensure curtains closed. Encourage patient to do as much as they can for themselves during the procedure. Ensure that only the area being washed is uncovered, and that patient is warm throughout procedure. Ensure that patient is involved in conversation. Do not speak about 'what you did last night' over patient. Offer patient toilet if required. Ensure teeth and mouth are clean. Offer drink. Tidy up. Leave patient comfortable with buzzer, drink and ensure that patient has everything they need before leaving them. (Practice Development Nurse, acute hospital)

Source: RCN (2008a)

Dealing with the behaviour of colleagues

If you observe colleagues acting in a way that does not maintain privacy and dignity, first try to counteract their behaviour. For example, if privacy is at risk, depending on the situation, you could cover the person up, offer a dressing gown, help the patient to dress or pull the curtains fully shut. You could introduce a colleague (who has omitted to introduce themselves), involve patients in conversations (when colleagues are talking over them), offer explanations and information (when they are not offered), and ensure patients' consent and involvement in decisions, where absent. In some situations, you might apologise to patients for your colleagues' behaviour and aim to restore dignity by demonstrating compassion and meeting immediate privacy and dignity needs.

As well as direct action to restore privacy and dignity, you also need to consider how you might deal with your colleagues' behaviour. You could raise the issue in private, for example: *'Can I have a word?'* and take them to a quiet room to discuss the issue. You should focus on the behaviour not the individual themselves (i.e. avoid being personal), encouraging them to think about how it might feel for the patient to be in this situation. Try to be constructive, suggesting how their approach could be adjusted so that dignity is promoted. Where applicable, reinforce any positive behaviour which they showed.

If a colleague's behaviour is abusive, you should report the incident to your line manager. Record the details of the incident, ensuring that you write clearly exactly what happened and the people involved. If any of your colleagues' behaviour consistently lacks attention to privacy and dignity you should also talk to your manager. Your organisation should have a whistle-blowing policy to support you in reporting poor practice.

Care environment issues

You may feel that some privacy and dignity issues need to be tackled with your colleagues as a team You could raise these issues at team meetings, explaining how you feel these issues affect patients and what you feel needs to be done. Examples of issues to be addressed as a team include: insufficient staff and unacceptable workload, a consistent lack of laundry affecting patients' hygiene and comfort, doors that do not lock properly or ill-fitting curtains, the need for curtain clips/door signs, insufficient or unsuitable equipment, not enough staff to help patients at mealtimes, inadequate or inappropriate food provision (e.g. for specific dietary needs, religious beliefs), no quiet room for private discussions, or mixed sex sleeping accommodation and bathrooms/toilets.

Conclusion

Patients and clients' privacy and dignity must be maintained to ensure that they have a positive healthcare experience. Legislation, health policy and professional codes all support the expectation of privacy and dignity in healthcare. Many patients and clients are vulnerable to a loss of privacy and dignity, and care activities are often potentially invasive or intrusive. While the care environment and organisation influence whether privacy and dignity are maintained, the behaviour of staff when caring for patients has a major impact. Healthcare assistants must plan care activities carefully, with consideration to promoting independence and physical comfort. They should preserve environmental privacy, bodily privacy and confidentiality, and use communication which helps patients to feel comfortable, in control and valued. Where colleagues' behaviour or the care environment diminishes privacy and dignity, all staff have a duty to challenge and raise issues of concern on behalf of patients and clients.

Age Concern (2006) *Hungry to be Heard: The Scandal of Malnourished Older People in Hospital*. Age Concern, London

Baillie L (2007) *A case study of patient dignity in an acute hospital setting*. Unpublished PhD thesis. London South Bank University, London

British Geriatrics Society (2006) Dignity behind closed doors. Available from: http://www.bgs.org.uk/campaigns/dignity.htm (accessed 15th November 2008)

DH (2001a) *Essence of Care: Patient-focused benchmarking for health care practitioners*. DH, London

DH (2001b) *The National Service Framework for Older People*. DH, London

DH (2006a) *About the Dignity in Care campaign*. Available from http://www.dh.gov.uk/en/SocialCare/Socialcarereform/Dignityincare/index.htm. (Accessed 15th November 2008)

DH (2006b) *Dignity in care' public survey, October 2006 Report of the survey Gateway number: 7213*. http://www.dh.gov.uk/en/Publicationsandstatistics/Publications/PublicationsPolicyAndGuidance/DH_4139552 (Accessed 15th November 2008)

Great Britain (1998) *Human Rights Act c. 42*. HMSO, London

Health Advisory Service (2000) *'Not because they are old': An independent inquiry into the care of older people on acute wards in general hospitals*. Health Advisory Service, London

Healthcare Commission (2007) *Caring for Dignity: A National Report on Dignity in Care for Older People While in Hospital*. Commission for Healthcare Audit and Inspection, London

Help the Aged (2007) *The Challenge of Dignity in Care: upholding the rights of the individual*. Help the Aged, London

Mencap (2007) *Death by indifference*. Mencap, London

Hlén J (2004) Violation of dignity in care-related situations. *Research and Theory for Nursing Practice: an International Journal* **18**(4): 371–85

Royal College of Nursing (2008a) *Defending Dignity: opportunities and challenges for nursing*. RCN, London

Royal College of Nursing (2008b) *Dignity: about the RCN's Dignity campaign*. Available from: http://www.rcn.org.uk/newsevents/campaigns/dignity (accessed 15th November 2009)

Social Care Institute for Excellence (2006) *Practice guide 09: Dignity in Care*. Available from: http://www.scie.org.uk/publications/practiceguides/practiceguide09 (accessed 15th November 2008)

United Nations (1948) *The Universal Declaration of Human Rights.* Available from http://www.un.org/Overview/rights.html (accessed 15th November 2008)

Woolhead G, Calnan M, Dieppe P, Tadd W (2005) Dignity in older age: what do older people in the United Kingdom think? *Age and Ageing* **33**(2): 165–70

CHAPTER 2

Communication and documentation

Angela Grainger and Ann Pegram

Communication is about either sending or receiving messages. The sender needs to be clear about what is being conveyed so that the receiver fully understands the context of the conversation or an instruction. Interpretation of meaning is therefore something that occurs between the sender and the receiver of the communication. Where the message is ambiguous so that more than one meaning could be interpreted any resultant action might be taken in a way that was never originally intended and mistakes can occur. This is an issue with verbal and written communications and therefore this chapter will address the required good practices in verbal, non-verbal (body language), and written communications. In this context written communications will be referred to as documentation.

Verbal and non-verbal communication

We often communicate with the patient and members of the care team verbally. A good overall benchmark is to remember to talk to or about someone in the manner that you would like to be addressed. If you think you would be uncomfortable or embarrassed with your mode of speech then work on changing your approach until you are satisfied that no offence can be taken. There will be a senior member of staff, and in some organisations, a staff development manager/teacher who can help with this if required. Many organisations have incorporated a set of communication and behaviour standards as part of their corporate culture. You should obtain a copy of these if compliance with these is mentioned in your job description. You should also receive training on these standards as part of your induction if you are newly appointed, or as part of your continuing professional development if you are already in post.

Always think about what you need to say, and take into account to whom you are speaking. Someone from a different cultural background might need something explaining in a different way or to be taken and shown where something is, for example, the toilet facilities or the kitchen. We need to take these types of issues into account when talking to patients, relatives, and colleagues.

Rapport and relationship building stems from good communication practices and is important in making patients feel they can approach and trust us. For healthcare professionals, good communication practices means that patients are more likely to cooperate with investigations and treatments, and also any on-going care upon discharge, including that which they might be expected to undertake themselves. This is because our communication practices have helped to enable them to understand what is expected of them and why. If patients and relatives really do not comprehend English then liaise with a senior member of your team so that an interpreter is obtained. Often other family members who do speak English will act as an interpreter, and there will often be staff who can speak that particular language. Most health care organisations maintain a list of contactable interpreters. In the event of real difficulty in obtaining an interpreter, the local police often have interpreter contacts. Be mindful of the laws governing confidentiality when asking somebody to interpret.

Other patients who might have particular needs in communicating are very young children, those who have a learning disability, patients who have had a stroke (a cerebrovascular incident) and who because of this have slurred speech, a severe speech impediment, or no speech at all, those who have facial injuries; and those who communicate in a distinctive way by either using sign language if they are hard of hearing, or Braille if they have no sight and have been taught to read in this way. Elderly, confused patients and those who have a dementia type illness tend to have short-term memory loss and therefore cannot easily recall what has been said to them recently. The healthcare assistant has to be patient and to be prepared to repeat conversations, sometimes many times over, in the course of a span of duty. Involvement of the parents, carers, and others who have a long-term significant relationship with the patient can help the health care team explain what is happening to the patient because people who know the child or the patient, understand what words or sounds are used to convey a particular meaning such as '*I want my special cuddly*', meaning a favourite toy, or a blanket, or a piece of cloth to which the child, or perhaps a learning disabled patient who is younger in mind than in chronological years, attaches a degree of comfort and security. Other phrases that loved ones can identify and which are of enormous importance to the patient, and therefore to the attending healthcare professionals in terms of the giving of timely effective care which also preserves the patient's dignity are '*I want the toilet*'; '*I want a drink*', '*I am going to be sick*', and so on.

How we speak and write are closely related so it is relevant to consider the overall principles of good practice relating to verbal and non-verbal communication because our body language often conveys a lot of meaning, not all of which is appreciated by those who see it. Sometimes we are not as aware as we should be of the signals our body language is giving out. These principles apply to all with whom you come into contact whether these persons are patients, relatives/visitors, or colleagues.

- Always maintain appropriate face-to-face contact. Do not stare but have an approachable, friendly manner. A smile, providing this is appropriate to the circumstances, is always a welcoming sign and indicates a feeling of '*I have time for you*'
- Speak to the person addressing you, or whom you are addressing. Do not speak over your shoulder no matter how busy you are. It is rude and dismissive and furthermore you cannot see the facial expression of the other person to see if they look puzzled, alarmed, cross, or upset. You cannot therefore easily adjust your next response to the other person's reaction, and thereby turn what might be becoming a negative situation to a more positive interaction
- Speak clearly and respectfully. Do not raise your voice. Just because someone does not seem to understand does not mean the person is stupid. Raising your voice and being impatient or irritated will not facilitate or hasten the understanding process. It will instead show that we have an irritated and impatient member of the nursing team
- Find out from the patient how he or she likes to be addressed. Do not assume you have permission to call patients by their first names. Do not demean people by using general endearments such as '*love*', *dear*, '*pet*' or '*ducky*'. It is generally considered to be an affront to a patient's dignity. It can sometimes signify that the healthcare staff cannot be bothered to find out from each individual patient how he or she wishes to be addressed. If a patient wishes to be addressed by us by his/her first name, or has a preferred name, then document this in the patient record so that all members of the team know. Documenting this also signifies that you are working in accordance with the spirit of giving individualised care
- Tactfully enquire if the information or instruction you have relayed is understood. If not, repeat the information and consider using additional ways of conveying the meaning. For example, show the person the piece of equipment being explained, and even demonstrate what has to be done with this and how it operates, or show where something is kept. If the person still does not understand then in a friendly way convey that this is not a cause for worry, and go and ask a senior member of the team to come and explain

- Do not allow your face to give away your inner thoughts. You might say you are not irritated by something but your face might show otherwise. The messages conveyed by the face should correspond to the message being conveyed by speech otherwise we run the risk of being false and being perceived as lacking integrity. Patients who have an altered body image can experience loss of self esteem and therefore look to members of the nursing team for continued acceptance as a normal human being, as well as for comfort and support. If our facial expressions inform the patient that we, too, find the altered body image distressing then this can severely hinder the patient's recovery and acceptance of the new body image. When managing the disposal of urine and faeces, which on occasions can be malodorous, control of our facial expressions has to be mastered if the patient's dignity is to be preserved

- Do not talk to people with your arms folded in front of you, a defensive, closed stance, or with your hands on your hips, an openly aggressive stance. Neither of these stances are conducive to people opening up to you, or to their wanting to engage in anything other than a superficial conversation. We run the risk therefore of closing ourselves off from our patients or their close loved ones who might want or need to tell us something of significance in relation to the patient's care

- Wear your uniform correctly and with a sense of pride in the service that you are part of. How we look and behave says a lot about how we feel about ourselves. Relatives of dependent patients do not have confidence that their loved ones will receive good fundamental nursing care in relation to the meeting of personal hygiene needs if the nurses attending them look unkempt and wear a grubby uniform

- Learn the art of being an active listener and of picking up what the other person is saying to you. What he or she emphasises in speech and how this relates to the story being conveyed reveals true feelings. The emphasis on certain words, or the points at which the person shows signs of verbal or non-verbal distress allows you to interpret the actual concerns and to respond to this or to alert the registered nurse that this person needs further additional support

- Always maintain confidentiality. Information from and about patients should only be communicated on 'a need to know basis', meaning that pertinent information is only shared amongst the staff directly involved in giving care to the patient. If a patient says that he or she is only telling you something and that it is to go no further then you have to make a decision as to whether what has been disclosed is fundamental to the patient's care. If it is you need to explain to the patient why this should be mentioned to the registered nurse in charge of the patient's care or to the doctor if it is a purely medical or treatment-related matter.

Often the patient is seeking an assurance that something which he or she feels awkward or embarrassed about will be handled tactfully and that confidentiality will be maintained. Encourage the patient to release this information personally to the registered nurse or doctor. If the patient declines and you think it is really important then inform the registered nurse that you feel the patient needs to talk privately about something, without disclosing any of the content of the conversation you have had with the patient. You may have to tell the patient that he or she is unfortunately compromising your position in being able to give holistic care and that it really is important that this information is disclosed to the members of the healthcare team directly involved in the patient's care

• Never discuss information relating to patients that can identify those concerned in a public place. This includes staff dining rooms, bus stops, shops, and your own home. If you need to record something you have learned about an aspect of patient care in a reflective practice document or a learning log for continuing professional development purposes or to meet the requirements of an NVQ assessment then refer to the patient as Mr. X or Patient A, or by using a similar non-identifiable descriptor. This also applies to any members of staff with whom you have had an enlightened conversation and therefore gained further learning.

It is by conversing with patients and their relatives that we get to know what is important to them, what aspects of care they appreciate, or how they would like certain aspects of care delivered differently. Perhaps it is that they do not understand their condition and treatment and would therefore like a further explanation or are seeking additional reassurance. By interpreting what our patients seek from us accurately we are in more of a position to address their needs. Although issues significant to the patient's care might become apparent to us in conversations we have to have a way of ensuring continuity of care provision and act on matters of importance. Recording these significant issues, following discussion with a registered nurse, is where we need good documentation skills. When we remember how many patients each one of us cares for at any one time, and the complex care packages and treatment regimes many patients have, reliance on memory, and verbal communication skills, either our own or that of colleagues, is an insufficient mechanism for ensuring continuity of safe patient care. Most importantly we need to take note of the subtle and early adverse changes in the patient's condition so that any required corrective action is taken to try and prevent any further deterioration in the patient's health. By noticing things and following up on them your patients are safe, and you are fulfilling your expected duties in a conscientious way. Being observant and conscientious are core skills of any nursing role.

Documentation

Documentation is an essential element of patient care. In hospitals and in certain residential care settings there is a nursing, or paid carer presence provided throughout each 24 hours of the 7 days of the week, and in the various community settings, including the patient's own home, regular visiting care might be being provided. However, it is never the same nurse or carer involved every time in the delivery of that care, irrespective of the setting. We work in teams and on a shift-by-shift or rota basis, and so we can only give individualised and holistic care to patients if the patient's assessment of care and on-going needs is communicated and shared amongst all the team members. Remember that the members of the team include the patient, who is central to the team, and his or her family members or any others with whom the patient has a significant relationship. Without input and feedback from the patient, or from someone who knows the patient and whom the patient trusts to speak on his or her behalf, our assessment of the patient's continuing care needs and the plan of care designed to meet these needs, however professionally and competently done, will be inadequate in terms of fulfilling the spirit of care-giving in accordance with knowing how the patient feels about this.

It is essential to document key aspects of care in the patient's care plan in accordance with the documentation policy of your employing organisation because otherwise essential elements of care can be overlooked with damage resulting to the patient. From an evidential point of view, if a serious complaint is made, or a legal case is taken up, it is more difficult to demonstrate that care was given when it has not in fact been documented. The safety valve saying that most professional health care workers live by is '*If you've done it, document it*'.

The purpose of documentation is to enable effective communication between the various members of the multi-professional healthcare team involved in the patient's care, to reduce risk of errors and damage resulting to the patient, and to maintain continuity of care. Accurate and timely documentation is acknowledged as being a crucial aspect of the role of the registered nurse (Nursing and Midwifery Council [NMC], 2008). As a care assistant one of your key responsibilities will be assisting the registered nurse in the preparation of documents associated with patient care and the updating of patient records. To achieve good record keeping it is important that you have an understanding of the key principles that underpin documentation.

Key principles of documentation

The Department of Health [DH] (2001) identifies that accurate documentation is essential for evaluating patient care, and therefore of the quality of care planned and given. The NMC (2008) identifies that a registered nurse must '*...provide a high standard of care of practice and care at all times*' this can be ensured by keeping '*clear and accurate records*'. Clear and accurate records ensure that continuity of care is maintained, meaning what aspects of care need to given when, how, and by whom. The keeping of clear and accurate records also needs to be considered along with other fundamentals that underpin care, for example the maintaining of confidentiality, how the patient record is stored, and who can access the record. As a general rule, a patient does have the right to access his or her medical record, including the nursing notes, provided the required procedure for requesting this is followed. As we have discussed above, patients need to be involved in the planning and the giving of their care so on some occasions patients co-complete the care plan with the nursing staff and therefore write in the record.

Clear and accurate records

The NMC (2007) issued guidelines on record keeping for the registered nurse to ensure that their record keeping is clear and accurate. Healthcare assistant can learn much from these guidelines in relation to how their own documentation should be made. The NMC identifies this can be achieved through records being completed at the time of care delivery, or completed shortly after an episode of care. Entries must be consecutive.

The type of care delivered can vary depending on how ill the patient is, but an account of the care interaction must reflect the event/outcome as it happened, or be completed shortly after the event. The record cannot be written retrospectively (meaning that a long time has elapsed after the event before entries were made). This also means that you cannot add anything to an existing record, or start to compile a record once a complaint has been made or a legal case commenced. This is to ensure that a full and thorough investigation takes place of what actually happened at the time and that there is no contamination of the existing evidence. It is recognised that for evidential purposes if care is not recorded it is deemed to have not been given (Dimond 2004).

When reading a patient's plan of care or when reviewing records it must be clear as to what the process of care was at any particular time. For example, who gave what specific aspects of care and at what time, and what was the outcome. The decisions taken regarding what aspects of care should be delivered, when, and by whom has to be underpinned by evidence-based knowledge which is why a registered nurse who is specifically educated for this will lead on care planning. Often care planning takes account of clinical observations and recordings such as temperature, pulse, respiration rate, and blood pressure, which inform us how the patient is physiologically and whether he or she is responding to treatment, and will also include observations of how the patient is feeling based on conversations the nursing staff have had with the patient or a close relative.

How often and when documentation is recorded depends on the patient's condition, where the patient is on the journey through the healthcare system, the context of care, and the nature of the record. For example, patients in an intensive care environment will have frequent observations taken and regular documentation made and a healthcare assistant might well be involved in this, whereas a patient attending a GP surgery or a hospital outpatients' department might only require the healthcare assistant to document the patient's blood pressure or weight.

Remember that the overall purpose of a documented record is that any member of the multidisciplinary team knows what is happening to a patient and gain a clear impression of the unfolding overall clinical scenario in terms of whether the patient's condition is stable, deteriorating or improving.

Records not being altered

If it is necessary to make an alteration to a record, then none of the original wrong entry can be obliterated or rubbed out. Any ink erasing products must not be used. A visible horizontal line must be put through the entry with *ERROR* written either above the entry if there is room, or alongside it, or just below it. The *ERROR* message must be clearly seen to relate to the line-crossed documentation. The person making the original error must then sign and print their name and job position next to the flagged up error message.

Records must be clear, legible, timed, dated and signed

All records must be easily readable, dated and signed by the practitioner. Registered nurses have a responsibility to countersign student nurse records entries if documentation has been delegated to students working under their clinical supervision. The time the care was delivered should be noted. Healthcare assistants might need to have their documentation countersigned by a registered nurse. This will depend on the documentation policy of the employing organisation. Factors that are likely to be taken into account are the type and level of documentation, and this will directly relate to the overall condition of the patient. If a healthcare assistant is working in a very acute or intensive situation it is likely that the registered nurses will undertake the documentation of the nursing care plan, and the evaluation of this in the patient record in line with their professional accountability. Whether the healthcare assistant has an NVQ Level 3 or equivalent qualification and has received further training on documentation and is working in a less acute environment are also factors that the healthcare assistant's line managers will take into account. The main guiding principle is that in the case of shared records the entry must be clearly attributable to the registered nurse who has been involved in the care. If a healthcare assistant is unclear about whether he or she has the authority to make a documented entry then the best course of action is to ask someone senior.

Records have to be factual

Records should reflect the type and standard of care given. It must not be based on the subjective values of the care givers. In hospital settings, it is now often the case that the matron carries out regular quality ward rounds in order to audit standards of care and the accurate identification of patients' needs. Part of the quality ward round is reviewing patients' care plans, the clinical observation sheets, and the patients' records in order to see that the required care is actually given and reflected in the documentation. Abbreviations should not be used as these can be ambiguous and therefore open to differing interpretations. An example of this is *MI*. *MI* can mean myocardial infarction (a heart attack), mitral incompetence (a faulty heart valve), or *MI* is an abbreviation for management information. Not all abbreviated meanings can be deduced from the context of care.

The account of the episode of care should be made explicitly clear. Phrases such as '*all care given*', '*up and about*', and '*self caring*' should be avoided. A description as to what is meant needs to be recorded. An example would be: '*Patient ate breakfast. Got up unaided and walked to the shower room, where he/she bathed him/herself without assistance*'.

The amount or volume of what is written is not the crucial issue. Accuracy and clarity are what is important.

Maintaining confidentiality

Whilst registered nurses are accountable for maintaining the confidentiality of the content of patient records for those in their care (NMC, 2007) — and this includes not only the content of the documentation but also ensuring controlled access to the record — non-registered staff are also responsible to their employing organisation for this in relation to their conduct. Your employing organisation will have a policy and a procedure on record keeping and access to records, including safe storage. You should familiarise yourself with this. Some organisations keep the patient record when not in active use at ward level in a locked notes trolley, with the nurse-in-charge holding the key. Procedures are also laid down for the sending and receiving of faxed information that contains personal patient information. In line with the 'need to know' way of working, dedicated and safe fax numbers are used in order to maintain confidentiality. With the advent of electronic patient records (EPR) access to the computer via an authorised password may be restricted to key care givers. If you are required to make statement entries on an EPR system you need to receive appropriate training on this from your employing organisation.

Patient involvement in record keeping

Patient involvement is a crucial part of nursing care. The NMC (2007) identifies that it is an essential criterion of good practice in record keeping to be able to see from the documentation that patients are, wherever possible, actively involved in their care planning. When involving patients or clients in their care we should identify how the patients/clients would prefer care to be delivered, and again where possible, under what circumstances. Good practice in documentation includes the following:

- Write in black ink as this is more durable. In the event of a complaint needing to be investigated, or documentation needing to be released in the event of a legal case, black ink entries make for better photocopying
- Write legibly, and act upon what you have written
- Be clear and concise in what you are saying and therefore writing. Concentrate on what the message is that you have to convey
- Date and sign everything. If it is important to give a time for when something significant happened then do so. Use the 24 hour clock
- Be factual. Do not embellish. Your personal opinions are just that, personal opinions. What is required is a succinct summary, professionally expressed, of what care has been planned for the patient and how this care has been delivered and whether this has met the needs of the patient
- Use neutral and politically correct language in order to avoid being offensive. Personal remarks about a person's cultural background, skin colour, gender, sexual orientation, and the presence of a disability, whether visible or invisible, are unmerited and unwanted. If you are not sure what to document when a challenging circumstance has occurred, for example, a visitor arrives who is verbally abusive and who appears from the behaviour and the smell on the breath to be inebriated (drunk), then consult the registered nurse about how to express this is documentation. An example would be: '*An adult male visitor who stated he is the partner of B arrived on the ward at 09:00am on 20th February 2009. The visitor appeared to be unsteady on his feet, and there was a distinctive smell on the breath (?alcohol). The visitor appeared verbally abusive and said XXXXX.*' Remember to date and sign this statement.

You should print your name alongside your signature
- Read back what you have written to ensure that it is what you mean to say. A good test is to think if you would understand what you have just written if you were someone else and had not just written it
- If you have written something in error then follow, as explained previously, the correct horizontal one line score-through procedure for identifying and marking an error.

Adverse incident or accident forms

If you are completing an adverse incident or accident form then you should answer all of the questions asked by completing the appropriate text box where the written details of what occurred is to be made, or by ticking the appropriate answer if some option responses are present on the form. Do not leave any blanks. If something is not applicable then state this in the appropriate response section. Please note that you should only be completing such forms if you were present, or on duty nearby when the adverse incident or accident occurred. This cannot be delegated to you to do retrospectively by someone who was present but who omitted to complete the required form at the time. These forms can be used for legal purposes so they must be completed appropriately and accurately.

If you are asked by your manager for a statement in relation to an incident or a complaint, or because you have witnessed an incident, then think about what you need to say in a logical fashion keeping the train of events and the sequence of things clear and in chronological order. Be honest and accurate in what you say. Date and sign your statement. There are reasonable and expected timeframes for you to respond to such a request. For example for written NHS complaints managers are expected to respond with a reply within 21 days of receipt of the complaint, so please do not delay in giving your statement to the manager. If you are a member of a union or a professional association, you can, of course, ask a representative of this to go through your statement with you before you submit it.

Conclusion

By following the key principles outlined in this chapter in relation to good practice in communication, and documentation in particular, patients are assured of safe care designed to meet their specific needs. It is both time consuming and upsetting to try and put things right when things have gone wrong, rather than doing things correctly in the first place. By getting communication and documentation right from the very beginning by adhering to the expected standards, healthcare professionals minimise the risk of being involved in mistakes or complaints.

DH (2001) *The Essence of Care: patient-focused benchmarking for health care practitioners.* Stationery Office, London

Dimond BC (2004) *Legal Aspects of Nursing.* Pearson Education Limited, London

NMC (2007) Record Keeping. Nursing & Midwifery Council, London

NMC (2008) The Code — Standards of Conduct; Performance and Ethics for Nurses and Midwives. Nursing & Midwifery Council, London

CHAPTER 3

The importance of clinical observations

Angela Grainger

Most healthcare assistants are required to take and record a patient's clinical observations, by which is meant temperature, pulse, respirations, and blood pressure. As these observations are part of the overall picture of the patient's clinical condition, which medical staff rely on to assist in establishing a diagnosis and to see whether the patient's condition is improving or deteriorating, it is important to be conscientious and accurate.

Healthcare assistants often spend long periods of time giving direct care to patients and are therefore in a good position to observe their patients and to get to know them in terms of how they are physically, and also how they are feeling. These more general, but nevertheless focused observations, are as important as the recording of clinical observations. Both sets of observations tend to inform each other, by which is meant that a more complete picture of the overall condition of the patient is obtained when you compare the clinical observations recordings with how the patient looks and how the patient says he/she is feeling.

Why accuracy is important

Accurate recordings of the clinical observations of temperature, pulse, respirations, and blood pressure give, over time, a pattern of physiological activity which can then be interpreted by medical and registered nursing staff in terms of any causative mechanisms. An example of this in an adult setting could be where a patient who has limited mobility has a slight rise in temperature (37.2–37.5°C) for a couple of days and then complains of calf pain. The inflammatory response of a blood clot forming in a vein of the lower limb (a deep vein thrombosis or DVT) has led to an increase in body temperature.

As soon as a patient in a hospital setting has signs of being acutely unwell by having either an increase or a decrease in the normal parameters (accepted normal levels or boundaries) of any clinical observation, for example a high or low temperature, a fast or slow pulse, an excessive or a decreased respiratory rate, or a raised or low blood pressure, the registered nurse must be informed and the frequency of the recording of the required clinical observation(s) increased. For example, a patient who has a raised temperature will have temperature, pulse and respiration rate recordings taken every 4 hours, as will a patient who has a raised blood pressure, above 140/90 mmHg (hypertension) or a rather low blood pressure, below 100/60 mmHg (hypotension).

By accurately recording clinical observations we are showing diligence in putting patients' needs first by recognising that unless we pay attention to monitoring the patient's condition we might not recognise the early signs of physiological problems that lead to a deteriorating condition. Recording clinical observations is therefore part of physiological measurement. Whilst the nature of some conditions means that we cannot always help patients to get better, the sooner we spot the onset of clinical problems and report these to the medical and registered nursing staff, the more we optimise the patient's chance of recovery or minimise the risk of longer-term complications.

In the previous example, the detection of a DVT in its early stage illustrates this point. If a DVT is undetected and is not treated it can lead to the blood clot travelling to the lungs causing a pulmonary embolism (PE), which if large enough can lead to a sudden cardiac arrest (the heart stops beating) and possible death unless resuscitative measures are commenced.

Patients' clinical observations are also recorded in various community settings such as the patient's own home or the GP surgery. This might be an initial recording to check the patient's physiological condition to see whether the clinical observations are within or outside the expected normal parameters of temperature, pulse, respiration, and blood pressure at that point in time, or might be a repeat recording taken sequentially over a period of time — for example blood pressure monitoring on a monthly basis at the GP surgery to see if the patient is responding to anti-hypertensive (high blood pressure) medication. It is important to remember that the results of clinical observations are only indicative of what is going on in the body at any particular time. Any abnormal results, meaning deviations from the normal expected parameters, must be reported to the registered nurse, or to a doctor, and a repeat recording of the clinical observations will be required within a short space of time depending on the severity of the abnormal recording. Very ill, vulnerable and dependant patients rely on us to make sure they are seen by a doctor as soon as their conditions require this, and this is another reason why the recording of clinical observations is so important.

Practicing under supervision

Recording the respective clinical observations of temperature, pulse, respiratory rate and blood pressure are skills for which there is an associated set of competencies that need to be achieved. Practice is the key to perfecting the required competencies. To begin with you should receive a clinical demonstration from a registered nurse on the proper techniques, and practice under his/her supervision before you are signed off as competent to undertake clinical observations on your own. Recording clinical observations is important for monitoring a patient's well-being or for detecting physiological signs of ill-health, it therefore cannot be left to guesswork or for you to try and work out how a clinical observation can be taken. Such an approach carries a serious risk of error in recordings and also means the patient is likely to have a rather unpleasant and uncomfortable experience.

Acquiring the skilled competencies in the taking and recording of clinical observations begins in your initial orientation and training programme where you become familiar with the core aspects of your job role, or as part of your continuing professional development (CPD). Reading this chapter is not a substitute for practice under clinical supervision, but should be seen as an accompanying tool to aid learning and understanding.

Whilst some healthcare assistants will be expected to take and record blood glucose levels this skill is not covered in this chapter. This is because there is a range of blood glucometers from different manufacturers available to patients and to healthcare professionals and although these all have the aim of monitoring blood glucose levels they all function differently. As blood glucose monitoring in both adults and children must be especially accurate in order to avoid errors in patient management this is a competence which can only really be explained, taught and assessed in the clinical setting. Remember that legally, in order to avoid being negligent, we must follow the manufacturer's instructions when using any product or equipment and have the equipment regularly checked and calibrated for accuracy.

Some healthcare assistants will also be taught how to perform neurological observations such as checking whether the patient's pupils are equal and reacting to light, and recording the patient's level of consciousness in relation to a predetermined scale, such as the Glasgow Coma Scale. However, these are likely to be NVQ/SVQ Level 3 healthcare assistants who are working under the direct supervision of a registered nurse in an intensive care or high dependency setting and who would be recording these after the registered nurse had taken these observations several times and the patient's condition is stable. The role of the healhcare assistant in this case is to assist the registered nurse, who would be doing particularly advanced nursing care on another patient at that time. This chapter does not cover neurological observations.

Observing the whole patient

Before we look at the basic physiological mechanics underpinning temperature control, pulse rate, respiratory rate, and blood pressure, we need to look at the overall clinical picture of the patient.

ABC — general first observations

A good starting point in assessing a patient's immediate clinical status is to think, ABC: airway, breathing, colour.

- Is the patient breathing normally, or is the breathing slow and laboured indicating hard physical effort in the act of breathing?
- Is the patient's breathing so slow and so quiet that it is hard to see that the patient is breathing?
- Is the patient's breathing rapid but shallow, and are the nasal nares (the fleshy side parts of the nose) visibly moving in and out indicating that the patient is trying to taken in more oxygen?
- Is the patient's airway clear so that the respiratory rate appears easy and the patient, if able to talk, can do so easily? Partially obstructed airways have a distinctive sound that resembles a deep groan with a whistling sound on either inspiration (breathing in), or expiration, (breathing out). Asthmatic patients usually have no difficulty breathing in but experience difficulty breathing out
- Beware the patient who has a partially obstructed airway who then goes quiet because this does not necessarily mean that the patient is getting better. A complete airway obstruction may have occurred, putting the patient into a respiratory arrest from which a cardiac arrest will soon follow unless the respiratory arrest is dealt with. This is also an important point to bear in mind when a patient has a tracheostomy tube in position. A tracheostomy tube is a surgical opening into the front part of the trachea (windpipe) which is inserted by medical staff for various reasons but the overriding reason for a tracheostomy is to provide and then maintain a clear airway (Dougherty and Lister, 2008). A patient who has a tracheostomy is not guaranteed to have a clear airway by virtue of a tracheostomy tube being in place, and healthcare professionals still have to check that the patient is able to breathe satisfactorily. Always look at your patients, not just at any equipment that might be attached to them
- Is the patient pale and/or sweaty? If so this could indicate a shocked condition? Shock is defined as lack of circulating body fluid and there are various causes for this. The reason that will most readily spring to mind is loss of blood through haemorrhage, but there are other causes.

Shocked patients have a raised and fast pulse rate because the heart is trying hard to pump some fluid in priority order to the bodily organs that need it the most, namely the heart, lungs, brain and kidneys. The skin is paler than usual due to constriction of the blood vessels. Dilated blood vessels cause the blood to pool rather than circulate and constriction of the peripheral blood vessels is an involuntary bodily response as a means of raising the blood pressure. Shocked patients have a raised pulse but lowered blood pressure

- Diabetic patients who are pale and sweaty and also agitated in manner may have too low a blood glucose level (hypoglycaemia). This is usually easily corrected by a small amount of a glucose drink being given but this must be done under the guided instruction of a registered nurse or a doctor. It is possible to over-correct the condition and to make the patient then have too high a blood glucose level (hyperglycaemia)
- Does the patient have a dusky or mauve hue to his/her skin colour? This indicates that the patient's cardiovascular system is being compromised. Observe the colour of the lips, which can turn blue, and in black and very dark-skinned patients observe also the palms of the hands and the soles of the feet as these can give an indication of the severity of the lack of circulating oxygen in the blood
- Is the patient fully conscious or confused and disorientated? If the patient is disorientated and/or agitated and has a dusky mauve colour this could indicate a lack of oxygenated blood getting to the brain. As the brain is one of the priority organs that the body tries to protect from the effects of lack of oxygen, an agitated but semi-conscious patient whose colour is turning a dusky blue is a sign that urgent medical attention is needed
- Is there any smell such as acetone or pear drops coming from an unconscious patient's breath? If so, the patient could be in a diabetic coma. Urgent medical attention is needed
- Is the patient able to speak easily? If so, the airway is clear, and the patient's cardiovascular system is not obviously compromised? If the patient cannot speak then he/she may have had a cerebrovascular incident (a stroke). It is important to keep a close eye on the patient's airway and to only offer sips of fluid once the registered nurse or doctor has assessed the patient's swallowing reflex or else the patient could choke and asphyxiate due to inhaling fluid into the lung(s). Always remember to talk to your patients and to be reassuring even if the patients cannot talk back to you.

Specific clinical observations

Before recording any clinical observations always introduce yourself to the patients, explain what you would like to do and obtain their permission

(consent) before undertaking any clinical observations. The only exception to this is where patients are unable to give their consent because they are unconscious or they have a significantly altered state of consciousness, in which case you will receive permission and instruction from the registered nurse in order to proceed. If the patient does not wish to have his/her clinical observations recorded then seek advice from the registered nurse. After completing clinical observations always remember to thank your patient.

Always wash your hands properly before touching a patient, and then again afterward before you attend another patient so that good infection control practice is maintained.

Never re-use single use products, for example aural (ear) temperature recording products. These types of products are designed by the manufacturers to be for single use and then to be disposed of.

Temperature

Body temperature represents the balance between heat gain and heat loss (Dougherty and Lister, 2008). The body's cells produce heat from cell activity (metabolism). Exercise and other forms of activity tend to produce further heat. Body temperature is maintained between 36 and 37.5 degrees Celsius (written as 36–37.5°C)

The main method used now for recording the body's temperature is a tympanic thermometer, which is inserted into the first part of the ear canal. This method also gives a reasonably accurate measurement of the body's core (internal temperature) as distinct from the body's outer or superficial temperature which can be gauged by touch. One of the reasons for the decline in use of oral thermometers is that patients often cannot keep their mouths tightly closed for long enough for an accurate recording so that only the body's superficial temperature is recorded rather then the deeper, core body temperature. The other reason is that oral thermometers contain mercury which is toxic if the thermometer is broken and the mercury escapes. If a patient cannot have an oral thermometer placed in the mouth then an oral thermometer can be used under the armpit (in the axilla) to record the temperature.

If you are required to use a mercury thermometer to take an oral or an axillary temperature then please ensure you are taught how to do this by a registered nurse. To record a temperature follow the instructions below

- Inspect the ear canal for any wax or rashes. Otitis media externa is a very painful condition and is where an infected rash with crustations forms on the skin covering the outer and the first part of the inner ear. In the acute stage the patient cannot bear anyone to touch the area so another method of recording the temperature is by use of a Tempa Dot (3M) on the

forehead, which is the thermometer technique mainly used for children. Wax can usually be gently wiped away from the ear with a moist warm cloth. Allow the area to dry before recording the temperature as otherwise the warmth of the cloth will influence the temperature result

- If the patient wears a hearing aid, use the other ear. If the patient has bilateral hearing aids then obtain the patient's permission to remove one of the aids for what is a very short period of time. Make sure you give it back to the patient or assist in re-inserting this as soon as the procedure has been completed
- Ensure the probe lens on the thermometer is clean
- Attach a new disposable probe cover
- Switch the thermometer on and wait for the ready indicator or the sign 'reading' to appear on the display screen
- Face the patient to show the equipment and then move to the side of the patient and gently insert the covered probe into the patient's ear
- Insert the probe cover so that the oval opening into the ear canal is covered by the probe.
- Press the activation button. Keep this pressed until the thermometer either blinks or makes a slight buzz (this depends on the make) as this indicates that the temperature has been recorded
- Gently remove the thermometer. Note the temperature recording. Document the result clearly and legibly in the patient record or on the clinical observation chart according to the practice of your employing organisation
- Note whether what you have recorded is significantly different to any previous temperature recording and if so report this to the registered nurse
- Remove the probe cover by pushing the eject button, which is clearly labelled
- Place the used probe cover in the appropriate coloured bag for clinical waste disposal
- Switch the thermometer off and place it in its charger.
- It is best not to insert a tympanic thermometer into the ear which is the same side the patient has been lying on. If the patient is having hourly turns it is probably best to record any clinical observations that need to be taken before turning the patient. If this is not possible then wait at least 20 minutes before recording the temperature as the patient's ear on that side will then have lost the heat generated by lying with that side of the head against a pillow.

If a doctor specifically requests that a rectal temperature be taken, then for safety reasons and to ensure the patient's privacy and dignity is maintained it is recommended that a registered nurse undertake this. Rectal

temperatures are now rarely taken so this is not a skill that a healthcare assistant can perfect by regular practice.

Pulse

The pulse is an impulse transmitted through the arteries of the body. The commonest site to feel a pulse is at the wrist on the palm-side of the hand below the base of the thumb, as this is where the radial artery runs. The pumping action of the heart causes the walls of the artery to expand. The wave-like effect of this is felt as the beat of the pulse. The arterial pulse therefore reflects the heart rate. The pulse can be affected by exercise and other activity, posture, and also emotions. The normal pulse rate for an adult is 60–80 beats per minute (Randle et al, 2009).

The main method for recording a patient's pulse is to locate the radial pulse and to count the beat for 1 complete minute.

- Locate the radial pulse which is at the thumb side of the upward facing palm of the patient's hand. Place your first and second fingers on the patient's wrist directly under the mound of the thumb and press gently until you feel the pulse beats
- Do not use your thumb. The thumb has its own pulse which could become mixed up with the rhythm of the patient's pulse rate
- Some older patients have a hardening of the arteries and this can make it difficult to detect the pulse beats. You may have to press just a little harder but be careful not to hurt the patient and remember that older people tend to bruise more easily. If you cannot detect a pulse and you think the patient has had a cardiac arrest then summon immediate help according to the procedure on your ward; if the death is totally unexpected in the home or in a residential care setting then make an emergency call to the ambulance service. Where the patient is talking and you just cannot find a pulse then ask the registered nurse for assistance
- Pressing too hard can also make it hard to detect the pulse rate; this is why practice makes perfect
- Look at the watch and wait for the second hand to appear on a clearly identifiable place on the watch face
- Feel the pulse beat and count the beats against the movement of the second hand
- When the second hand returns to the original identified place on the watch face, stop counting as 1 minute has passed, and the number of pulse beats counted in that time is the pulse rate
- Note also how the pulse felt. Is it a normal steady volume, is it thread-like and weak, or is it quite a fast and furious pace?
- Do not count for 15, or 30 seconds and then either quadruple or double

the rate noted to give the rate for 1 minute as this can hinder an irregular pulse being detected (Randle et al, 2009)

- Record the pulse rate and also any characteristics of how it felt on the patient's observation chart or in the patient's medical record as required
- Look at any previous recordings and note whether what you have recorded is significantly different in any way to previous pulse recordings. If so report this to the registered nurse or doctor.

Some patient's hearts may be beating at a rate that is different to that felt in the pulse. In this case a doctor might wish the patient's apex beat and radial pulse to be taken at the same time. A registered nurse will apply a stethoscope to the patient's chest where the heartbeat can be detected, and another nurse or a healthcare assistant will locate the radial pulse. The registered nurse will look at the fob watch and state when the counting is to start and will also say when it is to stop. Then simultaneously the registered nurse counts the apex beat and the second nurse or healthcare assistant counts the radial pulse. The radial pulse rate is deducted from the apex beat (the apex beat will always be faster because it is the actual heart rate heard through the stethoscope), and this gives the radial deficit. The radial deficit is then recorded on the patient's observation chart or in the patient's medical record.

Respiration

The respiratory rate is the number of breaths taken in 1 minute. The normal rate in adults is between 12 and 20 breaths per minute. Normal breathing at rest is a regular, almost silent rhythm, and is effortless.

- Maintain the patient's privacy and dignity and keep the patient warm
- Expose the patient's chest so it can be seen easily
- Observe the rise and fall of the patient's chest and abdomen. Each rise and fall counts as 1 breath
- Look at the second hand of the watch or clock and count the number of breaths taken in 1 minute
- Listen for any additional noises such as wheezing that accompany breathing, and/or whether the patient finds breathing an effort
- Note the rate, depth, and rhythm of breathing
- Record the rate and any other associated findings on the patient's observation chart, or in the patient's medical record.
- Look at any previous recordings to see if there is anything significantly different to report to the registered nurse.

Some patients' breathing patterns are altered as a result of being watched. As you get more experienced and skilled in recording these clinical observations it is possible to complete the pulse count and yet retain hold of the patient's wrist for a further minute whilst you then take the respiratory rate.

Blood pressure

Blood pressure is the pressure of the blood against the walls of the arteries. The systolic pressure (the higher level reading, which is the first sound to be recorded) is the pressure in the arterial system when the heart ventricles (the lower chambers of the heart) are contracting. The diastolic pressure (the lower level reading and the second sound to be recorded) is the pressure when the ventricles are at rest. Adequate blood pressure is necessary to maintain the flow of blood to the body's vital organs. High blood pressure (hypertension) increases the risk of a stroke, heart disease, and damage to the kidneys, and to the eyes (Randle et al, 2009).

Blood pressure can be measured manually or electronically. The general principles of electronic measurement will follow on after we have looked at the procedure for manual measurement.

- Allow the patient to settle before the blood pressure is taken. Activity can, for a short time, raise the blood pressure
- Remove any restrictive, tight clothing from around the patient's arm (the left arm whenever possible)
- Rest the patient's arm at a level that is consistent with that of the heart — Raising the patient's arm above the level of the heart will give a low reading, and having the arm too low will cause a higher reading
- Position the patient's arm with the palm facing upward
- Choose the correct arm cuff size. Make sure the cuff is clean in accordance with infection control principles. If the cuff is dirty liaise with either the registered nurse in charge of the ward or department or the surgery's practice manager so that a clean cuff is supplied. Generally, adults suit the adult cuff size supplied with the equipment but very obese patients might require an extra large cuff size. The cuff should cover about 80% of the upper arm.
- Apply the cuff smoothly and evenly. Wrinkles will increase the tension in the cuff and lead to a false reading
- The cuff will have an positioning mark which should be aligned against the brachial artery (the brachial artery is found just above the crook of the arm on the little finger side of the arm, and the pulse beat can be easily felt).
- Position the manometer column part of the sphygmomanometer so that it is vertical, at your eye level, and is within 1 metre of the patient
- Feel for the radial pulse and pump the bulb of the sphygmomanometer until the cuff inflates to the point at which the radial pulse can no longer be felt. This represents the systolic pressure

- Deflate the cuff and wait approximately 30 seconds, i.e. half a minute
- Place the listening side of the stethoscope to the brachial artery.
- Inflate the cuff to 30mmHg higher than the estimated systolic pressure which is when you felt the radial pulse could no longer be detected
- Slowly deflate the cuff and listen carefully through the stethoscope for two repetitive beats that follow each other in quick succession. This is the systolic pressure. Make a mental note of the reading
- Continue to deflate the cuff until no further sounds are heard. This is the diastolic pressure. Make a mental note of this
- Record the blood pressure on the patient's observation chart or in the patient's medical record, for example 130/80mmHg.
- Note any previous recordings and report any significant difference to the registered nurse
- If you are unsure as to the accuracy of your measurement then ask a registered nurse to recheck the patient's blood pressure
- Disconnect the cuff from the patient and make the patient comfortable.

There are different types of electronic monitoring and measuring equipment available so it is important that you are shown the correct use of the ones in use in your clinical area. Do not guess how the machines might work, or assume that one model with which you are familiar works in the same way as every other model. Legally we are required to receive instruction on every piece of equipment we use on patients and to be absolutely certain that we know how to operate the equipment before we proceed.

Some electronic and measuring equipment will record the patient's pulse, and blood pressure. The respiratory rate, and oxygen saturation readings are obtained via an oximeter, which is a finger probe which you attach like a peg over the patient's finger.

The following are general principles for when using an electronic sphygmomanometer for recording the patient's blood pressure.

- Allow the patient to settle before taking the measurement
- Remove any restrictive clothing from around the patent's arm
- Place the patient's arm so that it is resting at an equivalent level to the heart
- Place the correct size cuff around the patient's arm (the left arm whenever possible)
- Ensure the cuff covers 80% of the patient's arm and that it is applied smoothly, with no wrinkles or kinks
- Ensure the positioning mark on the cuff is situated over the brachial artery
- Press the start button

- Record the reading when any lights have finished flashing and the systolic and diastolic figures are shown as a steady reading
- Record the reading on the patient's observation chart or in the patient's medical record
- Note any significant changes from previous recordings and report these to the registered nurse or doctor
- Remove the cuff. Ensure the patient is comfortable
- Return the electronic sphygmomanometer to the place where it is kept. This is important in case it is needed by someone else in an emergency
- If a complete monitoring and measuring piece of equipment is used, i.e. a piece of equipment that will measure both pulse and blood pressure, remember to return this to where it is kept and also remember to re-plug it into the mains so that it will always have sufficient charge to be ready for use. Failure to do this can leave the battery flat just when you really need to get the patient's vital clinical signs recorded.

Other clinical observations that you will record are urinalysis, and the a patient's weight and height.

Recording urinalysis

A dip-stick test of a patient's urine can give an indication of what physiological problems the patient might be experiencing. Protein should not normally be found in urine. Protein in the urine usually indicates either a urinary tract infection or some other renal problem. Sugar should not be present except in patients who have diabetes mellitus. Acetone is found in patients who are not eating, or whose cell metabolism is impaired. Blood is present if there is a renal infection or other renal problems. Urinary Ph reflects how acidic or alkaline the urine is. Testing a patient's urine is a basic fundamental competence, the importance of which should not be underestimated.

- Explain to the patient that you need him/her to pass some urine
- If the specimen of urine required from the patient does not have to be a 'mid stream' specimen ask the patient to either go to the toilet and to hold the urine collecting container under the opening to the urethra (the opening where the urine flows from out of the body) so that urine is caught in the collecting pot
- If the patient feels he/she cannot easily do this, then place the pot in a bedpan and sit the bedpan over the toilet seat. If the patient is immobile then place the pot in a bedpan or in a commode chair if the patient can use a commode and ask the patient to urinate. The collecting pot needs to be nearer to the front of the bedpan or the commode because there is a greater likelihood of the urine being caught in the collecting pot

- If the patient is to supply a midstream specimen of urine then supply the patient with a sterile urine collection pot. Be careful how you advise the patient to open this or upon opening of it yourself. The inside of the pot must not be touched so that organisms on the hands of the operator do not contaminate the microbiological examination of the urine. Some collection pots are accompanied in their package by a wide necked funnel which makes it easier for the patient to use and to catch the urine
- Ask the patient to urinate a little into the toilet bowl, or into the bedpan or commode but ask the patient to also hold some urine back. The patient should then urinate into the collection pot, and thus provide a mid-stream specimen of urine
- Female patients who are menstruating and who do not have a tampon in situ might need to hold a sanitary towel either side of the urinary flow to prevent the urine being contaminated with blood.
- Put on your gloves (if you have been helping the patient you may already have gloves on) and collect the sterile specimen and pour a little into another unused collection pot so that you can apply a urine dip stick test.
- Make sure the mid-stream specimen of urine is correctly labelled with the patient's name, hospital number or other organisational identification, date of birth, and whether the patient is male or female, and remember to put the date and time of collection. The specimen should be sent to the pathology laboratory without delay, or in the case of the specimen having been obtained on a public holiday or during out of hours it should be stored in a clearly labelled specimen fridge until the next scheduled collection
- For the remainder of the urine, don gloves and dip one of the urine-testing sticks (after making sure they are in date) into the urine so that the colour range of every section of the urine-testing strip is covered
- Wait for the time period stated on the instruction sheets. This is usually 30 seconds to 1 minute, and then check the colour range of each section of the strip, which is clearly identified as relating respectively to Ph, protein, sugar, blood, and acetone, etc.
- Record the results on the patient's observation chart or in the patient's medical record.
- Report any significant findings to the registered nurse or doctor.

Some female patients might be required to have the urine checked for pregnancy. There are many different pregnancy testing kits available and you should receive instruction in the one in use in your organisation and also on how the patient is prepared for this test. If this test is being undertaken in an emergency department it is not usually the role of the healthcare assistant to give the patient the result. If you work in another area of health care and you are required to give the patient the result then make sure you know who to contact on the patient's behalf if the patient is distressed at either a negative or a positive result.

Weighing and measuring the height of a patient

Some patients are quite sensitive about their weight and height, particularly their weight. However, it is important to record a patient's weight and where possible the height as it can tell us whether the patient is under- or overweight. Some drugs such as general anaesthetic agents and chemotherapy drugs are prescribed in accordance with a patient's weight and body mass index (BMI). The body mass index (BMI) is a calculation of body fat based on the height/weight ratio for adult males and females.

Other reasons for weighing a patient are to know if he/she is losing or gaining weight, or if certain prescribed drugs such as diuretics which help the patient to excrete excessive water leading to oedema (an abnormal or excessive amount of fluid within bodily tissues that causes swelling) is working. In frail elderly patients and for other dependant patients, knowing the patient's baseline weight upon admission allows us to gauge whether they are becoming malnourished over time.

BMI is a person's weight in kilograms, divided by the person's weight in metres squared. Luckily, we do not have to do the calculation because charts exist that do this for us. We only have to record the patient's weight and height and then align the readings to the point on the chart that gives us the patient's BMI.

- Ensure privacy and dignity. Avoid making any humorous remarks because patients who are sensitive about their weight rarely find such remarks funny
- If the patient refuses to be weighed then reassure the patient that the result is only shared with the doctor or the registered nurse on a need-to-know basis. If the patient still declines then let the registered nurse know
- Ask the patient to remove any shoes or overcoat
- Check the scales are at the nought or the neutral point before you ask the patient to step onto the scales or to sit on the weighing seat to ensure an accurate reading
- Record the result on the patient's observation chart or in the patient's medical record
- If the patient wants to know the result and there is no known reason why the patient should not be told then inform the patient of the result. Some medical staff have concerns about patients who have a known eating disorder such as anorexia being informed of their result, so if you are

in doubt about whether you should tell the patient to ask the registered nurse first. If the patient then asks for the result you can tell him/her that the doctor will be discussing this in the consultation
- Ask the patient to stand against the height ruler and record the height
- Read the results of the patient's height and weight against the BMI chart, which should be available in your ward or department, or in the practice surgery, and chart the corresponding BMI on the patient's observation chart, or in the medical record.

A person is considered to be underweight if the BMI is less than 18.5, of normal weight if the BMI is 18.5–24.9, overweight if the BMI is 25–29.9, and obese if the BMI is 30+

Conclusion

The overriding principles when performing any clinical observation are: to be conscientious about doing so; to be sure you have received sufficient instruction and supervised practice to be able to undertake the clinical observation competently; to record the results neatly, clearly and legibly; and to look back at the previous recordings to see if the observations you have taken differ significantly in any way because if so you must report this to the registered nurse or to the doctor.

Dougherty L, Lister S, eds (2008) *The Royal Marsden Hospital Manual of Clinical Nursing Procedures*. Wiley-Blackwell, Oxford

Endacott R, Jevon P, Cooper S (2009) *Clinical Nursing Skills: Core and Advanced*. Oxford University Press, Oxford

Randle J, Coffey F, Bradbury M (2009) *Oxford Handbook of Clinical Skills in Adult Nursing*. Oxford University Press, Oxford

CHAPTER 4

Infection control

Vinice Thomas

The purpose of this chapter is to give an overview of infection, the causes of infection and how it is treated and prevented. By the end of this chapter support workers will understand the unique and key role they play in preventing the spread of infection both within the community and in the hospital settings.

The Oxford dictionary defines infection or being infected as '*contaminated with a harmful organism or noxious matter*'. Most organisms such as viruses and bacteria cannot be seen by the naked eye and these are referred to as microorganisms as they require a special microscope in order to be able to view them.

We are surrounded by microorganisms such as viruses and bacteria. Some of these live naturally, outside of the body and some within the body; some are beneficial to man, but some are very harmful and can result in serious illness. For instance, a microorganism called *Staphylococcus aureus* is found on the human skin and will not cause any harm unless the skin is broken and the *Staphylococcus aureus* enters a wound or the blood stream where it may develop into an infection. Infections due to *Staphylococcus aureus* can range from mild localised infections to serious infections such as septicaemia and in some cases death.

The body requires the work of bacterial organisms to help create a healthy environment within the gut and the acquisition of vital substances such as Vitamin B and K. These natural organisms in the gut are known as normal flora or commensal bacteria. They are within their natural and safe habitat, however if they did not remain there they could be potentially harmful as they can cause an infection. Another example is the organism *Escherichia coli*, which forms part of the normal flora when it is found in the gut, however, if the urethra was contaminated by it there is a risk it could cause an infection in the bladder or other parts of the urinary tract.

When a virus or bacteria is harmful to man, they are called pathogens. This means they are disease-producing organisms. An example of this would be the rhinovirus which causes the common cold, or Group A *Streptococcus* which causes a sore throat. Other examples include *Salmonella*, which causes food poisoning. The severity of the disease produced by the organism varies depending on the type of organism and the health and condition of the individual. For instance, a young fit and healthy individual is more likely to make a recovery from a bout of influenza, compared with an elderly frail individual. Hence, an individual may be susceptible to an infection depending on their general health, the ability of the immune system to fight it, and the virulence of the organism.

Transmission of infection

There are causes of infections that are due to the patient's general health and condition, exposure to health care settings, healthcare staff, or healthcare treatment.

Direct contact transmission: this is the commonest means of transmission and is when microorganisms are transmitted on the hands of staff to patients, patients-to-patients, and patient-to-staff.

Indirect contact transmission: this is when microorganisms are transmitted from person-to-person from contaminated objects such as commodes, blood pressure cuffs, etc.

In addition, patients who are cared for in a healthcare setting such as a hospital ward or visit a general practitioners' surgery may come into contact with medical equipment, furniture, furnishing or staff who have themselves been in contact with infections associated with the health care setting. For example, a stethoscope that has come in contact with a patient with methicillin resistant *Staphylococcus aureus* (MRSA) and may carry that organism to another patient if the clinician who uses it does not clean it appropriately between patients. In a similar way, if a nurse, allied healthcare professional, support worker or doctor caring for a patient who has infectious diarrhoea do not effectively wash their hands with soap and water and dry them thoroughly afterwards there is an increased risk the next client may be put at risk of cross infection.

The environment, healthcare setting, healthcare equipment and healthcare workers can all pose an infection risk to patients. Another specific cause of infection is commonly found with the use of invasive medical devices. These devices are inserted into the body to help treat or care for the patient. If a patient is unable to eat or drink, a peripheral intravenous cannula (PVC) may be inserted for administration of an intravenous infusion. Breaks in the skin caused by insertion of such devices can pose an infection risk particularly if the skin has not been adequately decontaminated beforehand or during manipulation/access, post insertion.

Droplet transmission: this is when microorganisms are transmitted by large droplet nuclei in the air, such as the common cold. The organisms are dispelled into the air with sneezing but do not stay suspended in the air.

The human body's protection against infections

The body can be exposed to infection via a number of routes, including the nose, eyes, ears, mouth, and broken skin. When pathogenic microorganisms such as bacteria, virus or parasites enter the body a common outcome is often an infection. Examples include sore throats, ear infections, food poisoning, and wound infections.

However, the body has been designed to combat the effects of disease-carrying microorganisms.

The body's natural defence barrier includes the skin, which acts as a protective barrier against foreign objects, and tears that wash away particles and germs from the eyes. In the gastro-intestinal system, the body has fluids that comprise of substances such as hydrochloric acid, which can destroy some of the harmful bacteria or organisms.

One of the key defenses the body uses is the immune system. The immune system is a complex system within the body which involves different specialised cells that react in the presence of invading microorganisms to prevent infections developing.

The immune system has the ability to recognise the pathogen and produce a substance called an 'antibody cell', which is able to fight the pathogen should it reappear in the body at a later stage. In order to do this effectively, the immune system will multiply the antibody cell so that there are a number of them able to fight against the invading microorganism.

Unfortunately, there are times when the body's natural defense mechanism is insufficient and additional assistance, often in the form of antibiotics, is required to recover from an infection.

Management and prevention of infections

Medical treatments for infections often rely on the use of antibiotics or antiviral/antifungal agents. These medications are used to treat a variety of infections. One of the important aspects of caring for a patient with an infection is to minimise the risk of spreading an infection to other patients, as well as to visitors and staff. This is known as cross-infection. To aid in preventing this, a patient may need to be isolated (which is discussed later in this chapter). In most cases, thorough cleaning of the environment, equipment and — most importantly — thorough hand hygiene will help reduce cross infection.

If required, antimicrobials to combat an infection are prescribed by a doctor and administered by a trained and qualified health care worker, such as a nurse within a hospital setting. However, other aspects of care are required to treat infections effectively and include:

General patient care

An individual with a systemic infection, e.g. when the infection is invading the local tissues or present in the bloodstream, is likely to have a change in their body temperature, usually a high temperature (pyrexia), though in some cases they may feel hot or cold to touch. It is important the patients are monitored and kept as comfortable as possible. This can be achieved by regulating the room temperature or the use of fan/cooling therapy and warming therapy as required.

Dehydration is another common problem a patient may experience. As a result it is important that the patient is encouraged to drink fluids to help stay hydrated.

The patient is likely to feel tired due to infection, and may need assistance in maintaining care needs such as personal hygiene, using the toilet, eating and/or drinking.

Hand hygiene

Hand hygiene is the most important activity necessary to reduce the spread of infection. This includes maintaining short and clean nails which are free from nail polish, as well as not wearing long sleeves, wristwatches, bracelets and jewelled rings as these do not allow for effective cleaning of hands. In the event of broken skin to the hands these must be covered with a waterproof dressing to protect both the patient and the health care worker from infection.

It is vital that hands are decontaminated before and after patient contact, within the immediate patient environment, and after contact with blood or bodily fluids. It is important to note that every healthcare worker must also decontaminate their hands before undertaking an aseptic procedure such as cleaning wounds and changing dressings.

Where gloves are worn as part of a procedure it is still necessary to decontaminate hands before and after the removal of gloves as hands can still become contaminated upon removal of the gloves.

Wherever possible, soap and water should be used to clean hands. Alcohol hand gel should only be used to decontaminate visibly clean hands as it can be ineffective if hands are soiled. When washing hands, it is recommended

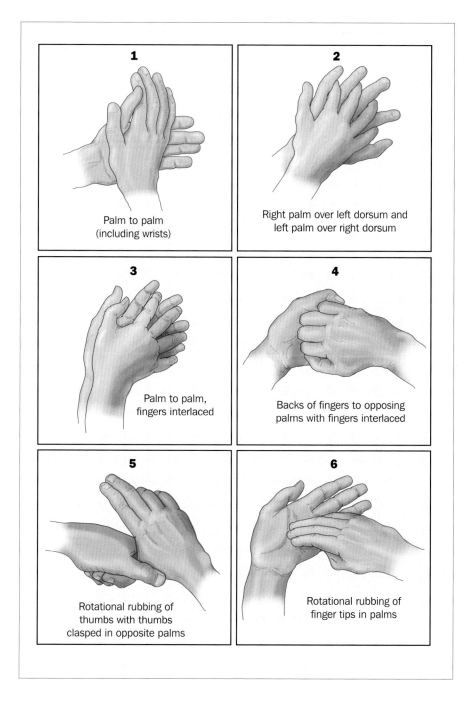

Figure 1. The six recommended steps to effective hand washing,

that the six steps of hand washing be followed on each occasion (see *Figure 1*). In caring for patients with certain infections such as *Clostridium difficile* it is important to use soap and water every time when decontaminating hands as this is the only effective means of preventing the spread of this bacteria.

Thorough drying of the hands is important once the hands have been washed, as wet hands are likely to lead to a transfer of organisms.

Personal protective equipment

Personal protective equipment (PPE) include items such as gloves, aprons, and face protection such as masks/visors and goggles. They are used to protect healthcare workers' clothing and mucous membranes and patients from cross infection and exposure to hazardous chemicals. In the hospital settings, additional items of personal protective equipment such as hats and footwear are worn, for example in theatres or the labour ward. The two most commonly used items of personal protective equipment for the healthcare assistant are gloves and aprons.

Whenever there is a risk of contact with bodily fluids such as blood or other waste products, or contact with mucous membranes or broken skin, gloves are worn to reduce the risk of contamination and cross infection. Gloves must be put on immediately before the task, removed, and discarded immediately after. Hands must be washed before applying gloves and after their removal.

Aprons are worn when giving direct patient care such as bed making, assisting with patient hygiene and decontamination of equipment or the environment.

In some cases, during an aspect of care, there is a risk of contamination of the eyes, face or mouth through splashes of bodily fluids. In such cases eye or face protection should be worn such as masks, goggles or visors.

Personal protective equipment such as aprons and goggles/visors must be changed in between patients and sometimes when caring for the same patient but undertaking a different procedure to reduce the risk of cross infection.

Decontamination of equipment

Within the clinical area there is a mixture of equipment that is re-usable, and others that are only to be used once and then disposed of; these are referred to as single use, or single patient use, equipment. Single use equipment must never be re-used. Such devices include IV-giving sets, disposable pulse oximeters and urinary catheters.

In order to reduce cross infection it is vital the correct technique and agents are used when decontaminating re-usable equipment. This will require that healthcare workers are familiar with the organisation's decontamination policy and have received the necessary training.

It is important that re-usable equipment, for example blood pressure cuffs, non-disposable bed-pans and commodes, etc. are decontaminated between patients. The level of decontamination will vary depending on the type of equipment. For instance, a re-usable bedpan will need to be cleaned and disinfected between patients, which will mean the use of moist steam to ensure any pathogenic organisms are destroyed. A bed frame will need to be cleaned and/or disinfected, which will require the use of a chemical agent.

Care of medical devices

Medical devices such as urinary catheters, nasogastric tubes and intravenous peripheral venous cannulae are used to provide support to patients during illness. However, the insertion of these devices can place patients at risk of infection if the device is not inserted under aseptic conditions and maintained using aseptic technique and constantly observed.

Qualified health care workers such as nurses insert these devices; however, it is likely the healthcare assistant will be involved in providing aspects of ongoing care relating to these devices. This care will include supporting patients with personal hygiene and ensuring the area around the device is clean and kept dry. It is important a qualified health care worker be informed of any signs of infection such as redness and swelling around the insertion site, or of any pain or abnormal discharge.

When caring for a patient with these devices in situ, care must be taken to ensure they are secured correctly and not loosened or dislodged when moving patients. Another example is the urinary drainage bag which must be correctly positioned below the level of the bladder to prevent backflow and not allowed to come into contact with the floor where it will be at risk of contamination. Healthcare assistants should ensure these devices are carefully positioned at all times. Any signs of dislodgment must be reported immediately.

Disposal of waste

Healthcare organisations will have a written policy on how to safely dispose of wastes, including bodily fluids and chemical spillage. This will also include the colour coding of bags used for the segregation of waste, e.g. black bags for domestic waste. It is vital that healthcare assistants are familiar with national colour coding policies and apply them correctly and consistently. Personal protective equipment should also be worn when handling waste.

Isolation

In order to reduce the likelihood of cross infection in some cases it is important the patient is isolated from other patients and visitors. The healthcare assistant will need to follow strict isolation guidelines around hand hygiene, the use of personal protective equipment, and decontamination of equipment and patient bed area and the general environment in these instances. Relatives and visitors must be informed of the procedure in a manner that preserves patient dignity, self-esteem and confidentiality. Where necessary, any queries about isolation may need to be referred to qualified healthcare workers.

The use of an isolation room will require signage placed appropriately to indicate that isolation is in progress. There is a need also to ensure doors are kept closed to prevent the risk of cross infection.

When providing care for the patient it is important that the necessary equipment and materials are gathered before entering the isolation area and that necessary assistance from fellow health care workers is arranged beforehand. This will reduce 'traffic' entering and leaving the isolation room, thus reducing the risk of cross transmission of infection.

Patients can often feel lonely and anxious about being isolated therefore it is important to provide encouragement and reassurance. The principles of isolation can also be applied to isolating a patient within a community setting.

Training

It is important to receive support and education in infection control training. This should be provided as part of the induction process and followed by ongoing, periodic updates. Included in the training must be hand hygiene, decontamination of equipment, environmental cleanliness, as well as understanding of the organisation's policies.

Infection control in various health care settings

The principles of infection prevention, e.g. hand hygiene and the use of PPEs can also be applied to caring for patients with a community setting, e.g. caring for patients within the hospital, nursing home or a patients' own home.

In the hospital

The hospital setting sometimes poses specific risks to the healthcare assistant which can often arise due to the large volume of patients being admitted and discharged, as well as the large number of staff employed. It is important that support workers are appropriately educated, trained and prepared to work in this environment in order to reduce the risk of infection personally, and to the patients in their care.

Staffing issues

Before working within the hospital setting, as part of the recruitment process, the employee will complete a health care questionnaire that will be returned to the occupational health department as part of a pre-employment health screen. This will provide an opportunity for the employing organisation to determine the immunisation status of the worker. Where necessary, health care workers will be required to be immunised against some of the infections they are likely to be exposed to during the course of their work. Healthcare assistants are at risk of needle-stick injuries that may potentially expose them to blood borne viruses such as Hepatitis B, C and HIV. Pre-employment screening will ensure that necessary precautions relating to infection and its prevention are highlighted. Once in employment, it is essential that workers follow organisational policy in the event of exposure to infectious or hazardous substances. This may include immediate first aid in the event of a needle-stick injury, and the completion of clinical incident forms.

In the hospital setting infection control can often be led and monitored (primarily) by infection prevention and control staff, though it is vital that all members of hospital staff recognise their own responsibilities in preventing and controlling infection transmission. Each hospital should have a series of evidence-based policies and guidelines relevant to infection control that are accessible to staff and consistently applied. A hospital-wide training programme should also be in place which all members of staff attend during their induction and follow up with periodic updates. In addition, staff need to be kept informed of infection risks which may be specific to them. For example, staff working within a respiratory ward are at an increased risk of cross infection from air-borne pathogens. As a result, they should be taught the various precautions required to address and reduce these risks.

Patient issues

Approximately eight percent of patients admitted to hospitals are affected by health care associated infections. Because of these infections the patient is likely to remain in hospital for longer than originally expected. This is not only distressing for patients and their families, but can increase the length of stay in hospital and costs the NHS an extra £4,000—£10,000 per patient (DH, 2008). However, many of these infections can be avoided if correct infection prevention and control procedures and practices are put in place and followed consistently.

Clinical areas such as accident and emergency, intensive care units and acute medical wards are busy areas, often with high patient activity. As such, there is often a higher risk of cross infection therefore rigorous adherence to policy must be observed.

Admission to hospital

On admission to hospital and before certain procedures it is sometimes necessary that patients be screened to identify if they are colonised with Methicillin-resistant *Staphylococcus aureus* (MRSA), or have other infections (HIV or hepatitis, for example).

Patients admitted with diarrhoea should be regarded/treated as though they are potentially infectious and all healthcare workers must adhere to strict standard precautions including the wearing of personal protective equipment and thorough hand decontamination. Where possible such patients will need to be isolated in order to prevent cross infection with other patients.

In the event of an infection occurring because of cross infection it may be necessary in some cases for an investigation of the incident to take place. This will enable the healthcare team to identify what the initial or root causes were for the transmission of infection and to take any necessary action to prevent this from happening again. It is likely that support workers who have cared for the patients will be asked to provide information on their contribution to the patient's care. The aim of the investigation is an opportunity to help staff learn from an incident and to improve the application of care.

General patient care

The general principles of best practice outlined throughout this chapter should be consistently applied when caring for patients within a hospital setting. It is important to note that due to the increased number of patients, longevity, the use of invasive treatment, and advances in technology, as well as the larger number of healthcare professionals, there is a greater risk of cross infection from HCAIs in hospital settings than in community settings, but this does not mean infections cannot occur in the latter. As a result, it is vital the patients are protected from infection at all times by healthcare staff applying the correct procedures and techniques, at all times, within all healthcare settings.

Discharge into the community

On discharge back into the community, if the patient remains infected then a qualified hospital healthcare worker is responsible for informing any community workers as well as the patient's GP. Healthcare assistants will need to ensure that all patient equipment, the bed area and the surroundings environment are appropriately decontaminated according to local policy.

In the community

Infection control within the community will vary according to the healthcare setting. These may include the patient's own home, and nursing or care homes. The principles already outlined throughout this chapter can be readily applied to the nursing/care home setting, however when caring for a patient in their own home there are some key points to consider.

Within the patient's own home it is important that the healthcare assistant maintain appropriate use of personal protective equipment and keep a ready supply available in the event that these are not available within the patient's home. Some private homes have limited hand-washing facilities and the support worker must adhere to good hand hygiene practices despite this and ensure they decontaminate hands using soap and water and also have a supply of alcohol hand gel and disposable gloves for use.

Removal of waste from within the patient's home must follow the policies and guidelines provided by the employer, and segregation of, for example, infected linen into separate bags for laundering must be discussed with the patient and family or carer.

Appropriate decontamination of equipment is vitally important in home care as unlike hospitals the range of chemical agents used may not always be available. It is important the support worker is familiar with local organisational policy as this will outline acceptable agents to use to disinfect, for example, medical equipment in the home. Any chemical agents used to decontaminate equipment must be stored according to the Control of Substances Hazardous to Health regulations 2002 (COSHH) regulations (see later)

Legislation

There are three key pieces of legislation which outline the responsibility relating to the control and prevention of infections as well as general staff health and safety issues.

Health and Safety Act 1974

The employer is responsible for ensuring staff are provided with information, equipment, instruction, training and supervision as is necessary to ensure their health and safety whilst at work.

Relating to infection control, the employer needs to ensure that infection control polices are in place, there are accessible and adequate personal protective equipment supplies, and infection control education and training is provided. Relevant staff must also be aware of and receive training on decontaminating medical equipment and caring for medical devices.

The healthcare assistant, as the employee, is responsible for ensuring that no action on their part, including failing to carry out an activity, presents a risk to patients, relatives or colleagues. Where the employee has identified a health and safety risk then action must be taken to reduce these. For instance, if it is identified that staff are not decontaminating their hands and therefore placing patients at risk of cross infection this must be reported to their manager/qualified nurse. In addition, the employee is responsible for using any equipment provided by the employer and for attending nominated infection control education and training.

In the event of an incident or accident occurring employees are responsible for reporting this to their line manager and completing any necessary documentation.

The Control of Substances Hazardous to Health Regulations 2002

The Control of Substances Hazardous to Health regulations (2002) (COSHH), outlines the responsibilities of the employer and the employee in the handling of hazardous substances. These include chemical agents such as disinfectants and bleaches.

The employer is responsible for ensuring a risk assessment is carried out before employees undertake any work where they are exposed to hazardous or potentially dangerous chemicals. Risk assessment should be regularly carried out and any necessary personal protective equipment made available. Cleaning agents, disinfectants and antiseptics will need to be stored according to the manufacturers' instructions and used solely for the purpose outlined in the guidelines provided by the manufacturer.

It is the responsibility of the employee to ensure the controls put in place by the employer are applied and the use of any necessary substances is in accordance to local policy.

The Code for the Prevention and Control of Health Care Associated Infections - Health Act (Hygiene Code) 2006 (revised 2008)

The Health Act 2006 details an organisation's responsibility in managing and controlling healthcare associated infections. The Act provides an overview of the standards required by organisations to ensure the patient is cared for in a clean and safe environment. The Code (as it is also referred) lists infection control policies and procedures that need to be in place and emphasise the

importance of leadership, design of the environment, and the importance of evidence-based protocols in combating healthcare associated infections.

The purpose of the Code is to ensure health care organisations have in place systems to ensure all users of the service, e.g. the patients and relatives, are provided with care in facilities that are safe and suitable for purpose. The Code emphasises the need for good clinical practice to be provided consistently.

National infection control campaigns

Healthcare associated infections are a key concern for patients and the public. Infections such as Methicillin-resistant *Staphylococcus aureus* and *Clostridium difficile* have had significant coverage in the media. To improve the care provided to patients and reduce the incidents of healthcare associated infections, a variety of national campaigns have been launched to raise awareness of the issues and promote best practice. This section looks at some of these initiatives and the benefits they have had for patients and healthcare organisations.

Towards Cleaner Hospitals — Department of Health (2004)
In 2004 the Department of Health set out a strategy to improve the cleanliness of hospitals and to reduce health care associated infections. Several actions were taken to achieve this, including individual inspections of hospitals with a view to supporting them to improve their systems and processes, introducing a 'charter' for matrons, and providing an opportunity for other hospitals to share best practice with each other.

Since that time the *Towards Cleaner Hospitals* team has worked with over 150 Trusts across England. As a result, hospitals have been supported in taking actions to reduce avoidable infections. Actions include implementation of *high impact interventions* (included as part of the acute-focused healthcare associated infections delivery programme *Saving Lives*), and ensuring all staff maintain high standards of care for patients — especially those with invasive medical devices — that all staff observe thorough hand hygiene standards, and that thorough decontamination of equipment and the patient environment is monitored and maintained.

Cleanyourhands campaign — National Patients Safety Agency (2004)
The National Patient Safety Agency (NPSA) is an organisation that focuses on the safety of patients and provides national advice on how to reduce risks and accidents to patients and users of health care services. In September 2004, a national campaign was launched in England and Wales with the aim of reducing healthcare associated infection through effective hand hygiene

Table 1. Five moments of patient care where hand washing needs to be carried out	
Moment 1	Before patient contact
Moment 2	Before aseptic technique
Moment 3	After body fluid contact
Moment 4	After patient contact
Moment 5	After contact with patient surroundings
	Adapted from WHO World Alliance for Patient Safety (2006)

— hands are to be decontaminated through effective hand washing and/or the application of alcohol gel, as appropriate. The campaign emphasises that correct hand hygiene technique is important, and specifically at five particular moments in patient care as outlined in *Table 1*.

The NPSA *cleanyourhands* campaign provided posters, leaflets and training videos, and continues to support Trusts in organising roadshows throughout their regions. The campaign has had a positive impact on raising awareness, with a community focused aspect of the campaign being launched soon. This will involve primary care organisations, ambulance trusts, and mental health organisations across England and Wales.

Wipe it Out — the Royal College of Nursing campaign on Methicillin-resistant Staphylococcus aureus (2005)

The Royal College of Nursing (RCN) is currently one of the largest nursing unions in Great Britain. Recognising the importance of reducing healthcare associated infections, the RCN launched the *Wipe it Out* campaign. The initiative promoted excellence in care by outlining evidence-based guidelines on how to provide quality infection control care to patients. The RCN also provide leaflets and posters to enable staff to promote the standards of best practice further afield within the health economy. Through the campaign, the RCN called for 24-hour cleaning teams to clean ward areas, infection control training for all staff, and on-site laundering facilities for staff uniforms. The positive effect of this campaign has been seen in an improvement in cleaning services and staff training.

Clean Care is Safe Care — World Health Organisation (2005)

Healthcare associated infections are considered a global problem and one which requires urgent attention and action to reduce. With the goal of building global commitment to this issue, the World Health Organisation (WHO) launched its first Global Patient Safety Challenge *Clean Care is Safe*

Care in 2005. Similar to the NPSA *cleanyourhands* campaign, the WHO also placed emphasis on hand hygiene improvement and the importance of hand washing with soap and water, and ensuring alcohol hand rub was used in the decontamination of hands and placed within easy access to the patient. Although hand hygiene played a major role in the challenge, *Clean Care is Safe Care* also focuses on other aspects such as safe clinical procedures, and integrity in blood collection.

Conclusion

This chapter has looked at the meaning of infection and how infections can occur. It examined the body's natural response to combating infection and the general principles of care required both within hospitals as well as a community setting in order to prevent and manage infections.

This chapter also looked at the national drivers in terms of legislation around infection control and the national initiatives that have helped to improve patient safety and quality of care. Following these national and international healthcare associated infection improvement programmes, there has been a significant reduction in infections such as MRSA bacteriaemia (infection in the bloodstream) in England, and hospitals have been provided with the tools and resources to help sustain these reductions.

Patients deserve the highest quality of care, therefore it is important to note that infection prevention and control is everyone's responsibility and that a range of measures will help reduce the risk of healthcare associated infections. By following correct hand hygiene practices, thorough cleaning of the patient environment, correct decontamination of equipment and care of particularly invasive medical devices, the rate of healthcare associated infections can be reduced and these reductions can be sustained.

The healthcare assistant has a unique and key role to play in reducing these infections. Through application of the principles outlined in this chapter and continuing to develop personal knowledge through the training and resources available, he or she can make a significant impact in the prevention and control of healthcare associated infections.

The Concise Oxford Dictionary (1991) Oxford University Press

Department of Health (2007) *Clean, Safe Care, Reducing infections and saving lives.* DH Gateway, London: ref 9278

National Audit Office (2004) *Improving patient care by reducing the risks of hospital acquired infections: a progress report.* the Stationery Office, London

Health and Safety at Work etc Act (1974) Health and Safety Executive

Control of Substances Hazardous to Health Regulation (2002) Statutory Instrument 2002 No. 2677 Crown copyright 2003

Department of Health (2008) *The Health Act 2006*. DH Gateway, London: ref 9286

Department of Health (2008) *Saving Lives Tool etc*. DH Gateway London: ref 9286

National Patient Safety Agency (2004) Cleanyourhands campaign, www.npsa.nhs.uk

Royal College of Nursing (2005) *Good Practice in Infection Prevention and Control Guidance for Nursing Staff*. RCN, London

World Health Organisation (2006) *World Alliance for Patient Safety: Clean Care is Safer Care*

Recommended further reading

Department of Health: www.clean-safe.nhs.uk

Infection Control Nurses Association: www.icna.co.uk

National Patient Safety Agency: www.npsa.nhs.uk

Infection Prevention Society: www.ips.uk.net

Understanding the skin in relation to personal hygiene

Sarah Mackie

Having an understanding about how the skin works is vital when caring for patients and their personal hygiene. Maintaining personal hygiene and appearance is important for physical health reasons as well as promoting self-esteem and dignity. Healthcare assistants play a key role in ensuring that the individual hygiene needs of the patient are delivered effectively. This includes accurate assessment and documentation by the healthcare assistant, as well as good skills of communication. Everybody has the right to receive a high standard of personal hygiene care. This chapter will incorporate seven main themes following an introduction. These are:

- The skin and bed bathing
- The mouth and oral hygiene
- The hair and hair washing
- The nail and nail care
- Facial shaving
- Cultural beliefs in relation to washing and dressing
- Privacy and dignity in relation to washing and dressing.

Many healthcare assistants working in primary and secondary care will be providing personal hygiene care to patients. The dependence level of these patients and the amount of assistance they require will vary. Patients' personal hygiene needs should be met according to their individual and clinical needs. All patients should be assessed to identify the advice and or care required to maintain and promote their individual personal hygiene (Department of Health [DH], 2003).

The skin

The main functions of the skin are:

- Protection
- Regulation of body temperature
- Elimination of waste
- Sensation
- Formation of vitamin D (Rhind and Greig, 2002).

The skin is the largest organ in the body, and an adult has a surface area of about 1.5–2 m² of skin. Nails, hair and glands are also considered part of the skin (Waugh and Grant, 2006). These are described as the appendages of the skin. The appearance of the skin can reveal a lot about a person, it is an indicator of general health, age, how the body is functioning internally, and emotional wellbeing. The features of healthy skin are:

- Is clear
- Is an even colour
- Is soft and supple to touch
- Is moist and unblemished
- Has a good degree of elasticity.

Many factors also affect the health of the skin, these include:

- Nutrition
- Circulation
- Use of drugs
- The environment
- Hygiene.

Other factors that affect the appearance of the skin are:

- The ageing process
- Exposure to sunlight
- Smoking
- Poor diet
- Lack of sleep
- Skin condition such as eczema
- Spots or boils
- Rashes caused by an allergic reaction.

The skin may also become dehydrated, dry or oily. It may also be sensitive to extremes of weather or temperature.

Structure of the skin

There are two main layers, the epidermis and the dermis.

The *epidermis* has a protective function. It appears thicker in some areas than in others, it is thickest on the palms of the hands and the soles of the feet; these are areas that receive more wear and tear. The epidermis consists of layers of tightly packed cells (Waugh and Grant, 2006). There are typically four layers of cells, however in areas that are subject to friction there may be five (*Table 1*). The epidermis does not have a blood supply or nerve endings; it obtains all its nutrients and oxygen from the dermis. This is why the outer cells die away because they are too far away from the energy source of oxygen and nutrients, which are obtained from the blood. If the epidermis is burned or damaged it can mend itself. If this happens to the dermis skin grafting is required as the dermis does not repair or heal itself (Rhind and Greig, 2002).

The *dermis* is the inner part of the skin. It is firmly connected to the epidermis. It is made of special fibres, tissue and collagen that provide

Table 1.   The layers of the skin

The outermost layer	Layers of closely packed dead, flat cells containing a tough fibrous material called keratin
The second layer	The cells are dead and flat, but are clear in appearance
The third layer	A thin layer of cells, it is an intermediate layer where the centre of the cells begin to break down
The fourth layer	This layer acts as an anchor, these help bond the deepest layer of the epidermis to the third layer
The fifth layer	This layer is the deepest layer of the epidermis. Its cells lie close to the dermis, from where it receives its blood supply. It is here that new cells are formed
Source: Rhind and Greig (2002)	

support, elasticity and flexibility. Unlike the epidermis it does have a blood and nerve supply (Rhind and Greig, 2002).

Sweat glands

Sweat glands are found all over the skin, the most are found on the soles of the feet and the palms of the hands, armpits and groin. The important function of sweat secreted by the glands is to regulate the temperature of the body (Waugh and Grant, 2006). Sweat is a watery fluid containing electrolytes and some waste materials (Rhind and Greig, 2002). There are two types of sweat glands, eccrine and apocrine.

Eccrine glands are more numerous, their function is to cool the body and excrete waste materials.

Apocrine glands are less numerous, and are located in the armpits, the eyelids and pubic/genital area. Their secretions have a stronger odour, and are produced as a response to stress, hormones or sexual arousal (Rhind and Greig, 2002).

Washing and bathing

Attending to a patient's hygiene needs is an essential part of the healthcare assistant's role. Activities associated with personal hygiene include:

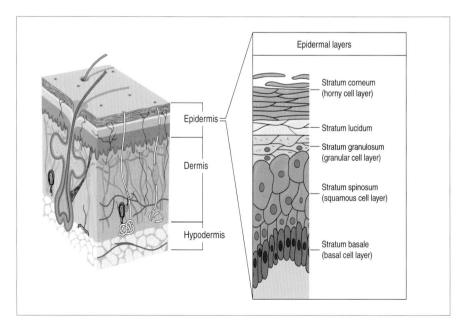

Diagram showing the layers of the skin.

- Skin care
- Showering, bathing or using the wash basin/bowl
- Oral hygiene
- Care of the hair
- Care of the nails
- Shaving.

Often these procedures are performed together, and the amount of assistance required will depend on the patient's level of independence and self-care ability. Awareness of interpersonal skills, including non-verbal communication is vital for effective care (Pegram et al, 2007).

If the patient has problems meeting hygiene needs this will be included in the patient's care plan, which will be written by the senior nurse. Patients may be totally dependent or only require minimal assistance. How much assistance is required may alter as the patient's condition changes, so care plans will need to be updated regularly (Yonwin, 2000). The care plan should indicate the following:

- The patient requires assistance with their hygiene needs, identifying their specific needs for example help with showering, oral hygiene and hair washing
- What level of independence is realistic for the patient, ensuring the goals set are achievable over a particular period of time
- Which areas of the body the patient requires assistance with, including particular lotions/creams/moisturizers that need to be applied
- Which areas should not be washed, for example wounds.

Bed baths

Bed baths can benefit patients psychologically, as they maintain self-esteem and help promote a positive body image. It also helps the healthcare assistant to build a relationship with the patient. This often gives patients an opportunity to discuss any concerns or anxieties. A bed bath is also a good opportunity to check the patient's skin for any abnormalities, soreness or pressure ulcers. There is a particular technique required for bed bathing. This should be used when a patient is confined to bed, or too unwell to provide his or her own hygiene needs (Doughtery and Lister, 2004).

For all procedures verbal consent should be gained from the patient and an explanation given. An experienced practitioner should supervise healthcare assistants delivering the care until they are competent and confident to perform the procedure independently. Also always ensure that universal precautions are followed and that the hand-washing and manual handling policies are adhered to.

The equipment needed for a bed bath is:

- Two towels
- Clean nightwear or gown
- Washbowl
- Soap
- Toothbrush and toothpaste
- Comb/brush
- Deodorant
- Disposable wipes/patients own flannel
- Moisturiser/talcum powder/make-up (if required)
- Shaving equipment (if required)
- Clean linen
- Linen bag
- Slide sheet
- Non-sterile gloves and disposable apron.

Prepare the patient by greeting him or her and explain the procedure. Wash your hands and put on gloves and apron. Two healthcare assistants should carry out a bed bath if the patient is unable to assist, one on either side of the patient. This will ensure that areas of the patient are not exposed for too long. Draw the curtains/screens around the bed, or shut the door and close the blinds if in a side room. Ensure the patient is covered with a blanket before the top sheet and night clothes/gown are removed as this maintains the patient's privacy and dignity. Ensure all the equipment required is within easy reach. Check if the patient has a hearing aid, spectacles and a wristwatch and ask permission remove these from the patient. The water should be hand hot, — if the patient is able ask them to confirm that the temperature of the water is suitable for them.

Washing the face
- Fold the blanket down the patient's waist and place a towel across the patients chest
- If the patient is able he or she may wish to wash their own face, ask if they use soap, pass them the wipe/flannel
- If they are unable to wash their face wash the eyelids first, then the forehead, the cheeks, the nose, ears and jaw, and finish at the neck
- Rinse the soap off the face
- Pat the face dry with a towel, avoid rubbing the skin
- Replace hearing aid/spectacles as appropriate.

Washing the upper body

- Place a clean towel under the patient's arm that is furthest from the healthcare assistant with the wash bowl
- Using a new wipe or the patient's flannel pass it over to the other healthcare assistant. This is to avoid any spills dripping onto a part of the body that has already been washed and dried
- Wash the patient's arm, armpit, hand, wrist and fingers. Check condition of the skin, and rinse off the soap
- Using the towel under the patient's arm, dry all the areas and repeat the procedure with the patient's other arm
- Remove towel from the patient's chest, so that one healthcare assistant can wash and rinse the chest, the other can dry the skin. With female patients particular attention should be paid to the area underneath the breasts. The skin should be checked for any redness, and ensure the area is dried thoroughly to prevent it getting sore
- Cover the patient with a dry towel or blanket and change the water in the bowl.

Washing the lower body

- Remove the patient's pyjama bottoms and remove anti embolic stockings if necessary
- Place a clean towel under the patient's leg that is furthest from the healthcare assistant with the washbowl. Cover the genitalia and the other leg with a towel
- Wash, rinse and dry the legs in the same order and method used for the arms. Check the pressure points on the heels and observe for any changes in skin condition
- Apply any moisturizer if required
- Before washing the genitalia ask the patient if they would like to wash this area themselves. If not wash, rinse and dry the area carefully. Use a disposable wipe or different flannel. If the patient has a urinary catheter, catheter hygiene should be carried out
- Discard gloves, wash hands and apply new gloves. Change the water in the bowl to prevent cross infection, ensure all wipes and waste are disposed of in a clinical waste bag as per local policy
- To wash the patient's back and bottom the patient should be asked or assisted to roll onto one side, away from the healthcare assistant with the washbowl. Appropriate moving and handling equipment should be used if required as per local policy. Care should also be taken with medical equipment such as urinary catheters, intravenous lines and drains
- Place a towel along the patient's back, wash, rinse and dry the back. Assess the pressure points such as the shoulder blades and spine, also

check the general condition of the skin
- Wash, rinse and dry the patient's bottom using a disposable wipe or different flannel. Check and assess the sacrum and surrounding skin. Discard gloves, wash hands and apply new gloves.

Changing linen and promoting patient comfort after the bed bath
- The healthcare assistant furthest from the patient rolls the soiled sheet into the centre of the bed (*Figure 1*)
- Place a clean sheet in the middle of the bed, rolling half the sheet up along side the patient ensuring the soiled sheet does not contaminate the clean sheet (*Figures 2 and 3*)
- Roll the patient on to the clean side of the bed, and remove the soiled sheet, and place in a linen bag. Tuck the clean sheet in, ensuring all creases are removed (*Figures 4 and 5*)
- Roll the patient back to the middle of the bed, put on patient's clean nightwear and anti-embolic stockings (if applicable)
- Position comfortably using appropriate moving and handling equipment as per policy
- Provide nail and hair care and oral hygiene as appropriate
- Apply moisturising cream and make-up if patient requests
- Place call bell within easy reach, and tidy away all washing equipment and linen/waste bags used (*Figure 6*)
- Remove and dispose of gloves and apron and wash hands
- Document care (Ambrose and Quinless, 2004; Pegram et al, 2007).

Oral hygiene

The main purposes of oral hygiene is to maintain a healthy and clean mouth, keep the lips clean moist and intact, remove debris and plaque from the teeth, limit or prevent infection, and keep the mucosal membrane inside the mouth moist.

A dry mouth can be a sign of certain diseases or conditions, and can also be caused by certain drugs or medical treatments the patient may be receiving. A dry mouth is caused because there is a decrease in saliva flow. Saliva helps to:

- Digest food
- Protect teeth from decay
- Prevent infection by controlling bacteria and fungi in the mouth
- Makes it possible to chew and swallow.

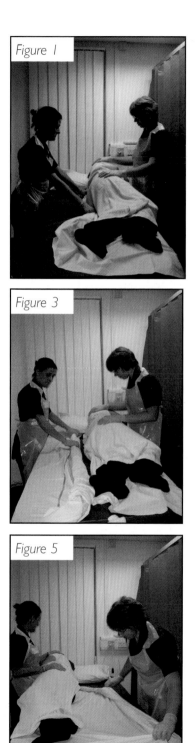

Figure 1

Figure 2

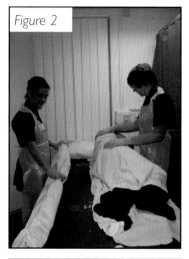

Figure 3

Figure 4

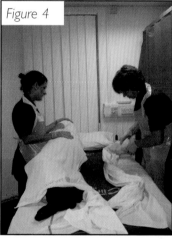

Figure 5

Figure 6

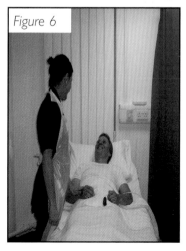

Signs and symptoms of a dry mouth:
- Sticky dry feeling in the mouth and throat
- Thirst
- Dry or cracked lips
- Problems with speaking, tasting, chewing and swallowing
- Bad breath
- Dry, rough tongue
- Burning feeling in the mouth.

Medical conditions and treatments that can cause a dry mouth include dehydration, anaemia (a reduction in red blood cells and/or haemoglobin), chemotherapy (treatment for cancer), diabetes, smoking, and oxygen therapy.

Treatment of a dry mouth will depend on what is causing the problem. Drinking frequent sips of water and sucking on ice cubes may help, as will avoiding drinks containing caffeine and alcohol. Doctors may prescribe artificial saliva or medication to stimulate the salivary glands. A sore mouth is usually caused by inflammation of the mucosa inside the mouth and/or ulcer formation. Conditions and situations that can cause a sore mouth include:

- Inflammation of the mucus membrane inside the mouth (stomatitis)
- Fungal infection in the mouth (candidosis)
- Poor nutrition
- Dental problems
- Poor kidney function
- Ill-fitting dentures.

Treatment of a sore mouth depends on the cause; this may include local anaesthetic sprays, painkilling tablets, locally applied painkilling gels and mouthwashes.

It is important for patients to clean their teeth or dentures regularly, in the morning and at night and following each meal. Any dry or soreness of the mouth, toothache or ill fitting dentures should be reported and documented so the appropriate action can be taken. If patients are unable to manage their own oral hygiene, then the required care should be carried out for them.

Equipment required for oral hygiene
- A small soft bristle toothbrush
- Fluoride toothpaste
- Plastic disposable cup
- Jug of water

- Receiver
- Box of tissues
- Towel
- Yellow soft paraffin/lip balm
- Non-sterile gloves and disposable apron.

Patients should be encouraged to maintain their own oral hygiene when possible. If the patient is able, take them to the bathroom to use the sink. If a patient is bed-bound a small receiver can be used under their chin. For patients who are able to sit in a chair it is best to stand behind them when cleaning their teeth. For patients who are bed-bound stand to one side of the bed.

- Greet the patient and explain the procedure
- Wash hands and put on gloves and apron
- The best device available for cleaning teeth is a toothbrush, with toothpaste that contains fluoride
- Use a pea size amount of toothpaste to prevent the mouth filling with froth
- Hold the brush at an angle of 45 degrees to the teeth (top and bottom)
- Move the brush in a circular motion
- Clean the gums next to the teeth
- Clean the inside surface of the teeth
- Clean the biting surface of the teeth
- The mouth can then be rinsed with water, however it is not essential as leaving toothpaste on the teeth will protect them for longer
- Yellow soft paraffin or lip balm can be applied to help soften the lips and prevent them from cracking
- Clean dentures with a toothbrush and toothpaste, always clean them over a sink with water as this will prevent them from breaking if they are dropped
- Document care
- If the patient is unable to rinse and void, use a rinsed toothbrush to clean the teeth and moistened foamsticks to wipe the gums and tongue. Foamsticks should be used with a rotating action so that most of the surface is used (Dougherty and Lister, 2004; NT Clinical Skills, 2003a).

Hair

The primary function of hair is protection. In humans, hair protects the scalp from sun rays and decreases heat loss. Eyebrows and eyelashes protect the eye from foreign particles. Hairs in the nostril filter the air we inhale. Hairs in the external ear canal also prevent foreign particles entering. The only parts of the body that do not have hair are the palms of the hands and the soles of the feet. The two regions of a hair are the shaft and the root:

The shaft is the portion of the hair that can be seen on the surface of the skin. The shape of the shaft determines the curliness of your hair:

- Round shaft = straight hair
- Oval hair = wavy hair
- Flat shaft = kinky hair

The root is the portion of the hair that is embedded in the skin.

Hair comes from the same tissue as the epidermis, and consists of closely packed cells that are made of keratin. In each hair (shaft and root) there are three layers of cells:

- The cuticle (outer cell)
- A cortex (middle cell)
- The medulla (inner cell)

Hair grows out from a follicle in the dermis. Attached to the hair follicles are small involuntary muscles, when these muscles tighten, they cause the hair to stand on end. This is often associated with an emotional response, especially fear. It can also be a response to cold conditions and is usually referred to as 'goose bumps'. The tightening of these involuntary muscles causes shivering-generated heat (Rhind and Greig, 2002).

Hair washing is another important aspect of patient hygiene that can sometimes be overlooked. As well as keeping the hair clean and preventing odour, it has a great effect on the patient's sense of wellbeing. It also promotes a positive self-image and can contribute to the prevention of infection (Baker et al, 1999). When washing a patient's hair the healthcare assistant should observe for and report any signs of hair loss/thinning of the hair, hair that easily breaks, sores on the scalp, excessive dandruff or dry skin on the scalp, itching of the scalp, infestation.

Hair may be washed in the shower, in the bath, at the patient's hand basin or in bed. If the patient is bed-bound their hair will need to be washed in bed. Equipment required:

- Two towels
- Jug
- Incontinence pads
- Bed-fast rinser (if available)
- Shampoo
- Conditioner
- Patient's comb
- A large bowl for water
- Bedside table
- Hairdryer (optional)
- Non-sterile gloves and disposable apron.

Bed-fast rinser - this is a large plastic tray with an edge that the patient's hair is washed over. One corner of the tray has a drip outlet; this enables the water to drain away into a bowl below (see *Figures 7* and *8*). If there is no bed-fast rinser available use the towel and incontinence pads to soak up the excess water. Ensure a towel is wrapped around the patient's neck, and always check if the patient has any lines in their neck or dressings. Care should be taken not to get them wet or dislodged. Patients who require their hair cutting should be referred to the hairdresser (Baker et al, 1999).

Procedure

- Greet the patient and explain the procedure
- Wash hands and put on gloves and apron
- Pull the bed away from the wall, and remove the bed-head
- Place bedside table behind the patient
- Cover the table with a towel and incontinence pads. If bed-fast rinser available place this on top

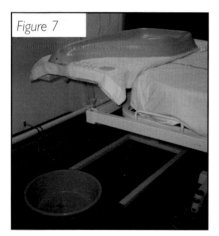

Figure 7

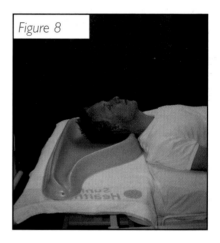

Figure 8

- Place jug and bowl of warm water within easy reach
- Help the patient move up the bed, so that their head is resting on the table/bed-fast rinser
- Wet the patient's hair using the jug
- Wash the patient's hair
- Apply hair conditioner if required, then rinse again
- Towel dry patient's hair
- Comb patients hair
- Move patient back down the bed, and ensure they are comfortable
- Dry hair with hairdryer if required
- Document care (Baker et al, 1999)

Nail care

Human nails are the equivalent to the claws, horns and hoofs of animals. They are made up of the same cells as epidermis and hair and consist of hard keratin plates (Waugh and Grant, 2006). In humans, nails protect the sensitive tips of the fingers and toes (Rhind and Greig, 2002). Fingernails grow quicker than toenails, and growth is quicker when the environmental temperature is high (Waugh and Grant 2006). *Table 2* shows the different parts of the nail.

Nail care is an important aspect of personal hygiene and grooming. When assisting or providing personal care for patients this also involves caring for their fingernails and toenails. Sometimes fingernails can become long, broken and dirty. If fingernails are not cared for then potentially the patient can cause damage to their skin from scratching, and the nails will look unsightly and they feel uncomfortable.

Equipment required for finger nail care
- Bowl of warm soapy water
- Disposable wipes
- Nail file
- Nail scissors/clippers
- Towel
- Hand cream (optional)
- Non-sterile gloves and disposable apron.

Table 2.	The different parts of the nail
Region of the nail	
The nail body	Portion of the nail that is visible, the nail body (plate) rests on the nail bed
The free edge	Visible portion of the nail that extends past the digit, it is the edge of the nail that you cut
The nail root	Hidden portion of the nail that is embedded in a fold of skin, the cuticle extends from this fold. Its function is to act as a seal and protect the space between the fold and the nail plate from external moisture.
	Source: Rhind and Greig (2002).

Procedure
- Greet the patient and explain the procedure
- Wash hands and put on gloves and apron
- Soak the patient's hands in a bowl of warm soapy water
- Wash with a disposable wipe and remove the dirt from under the fingernails, this will also soften the nail before it is cut, making it easier
- Always ensure the patient's hands are dried thoroughly
- When cutting or trimming the fingernail use a pair of nail clippers or nail scissors
- Ensure the nail is not cut too short to avoid causing damage to the surrounding skin and fingertip
- If required you can then file the nail using the nail file to create a smoother edge
- Apply hand cream if requested to help soften the skin
- Document care.

It is recommended that if patients require their toe nails cutting they are referred to a qualified chiropodist, unless the healthcare professional providing the care has received adequate training. If patients are diabetic they should be referred to the diabetic foot clinic, as these type of patients are more at risk of acquiring problems with their feet and may required specialised treatment. However healthcare assistants can still provide some aspects of the foot care.

If patients are unable to have a bath or shower they may like to have their feet washed in a bowl of warm soapy water; this can help them relax and also looks after the condition of their feet. Always ensure that the patient's feet are dried thoroughly especially between the toes. If areas are left damp the patient may be more at risk of developing infections or skin soreness. It may not be advisable for some patients to have their feet soaked in water, for example those who have foot ulcers or wounds on their feet or lower leg. Always check with the senior nurse and read the patient's care plans before performing the task. Providing foot care is also a good opportunity to check the patient's feet for pressure ulcers, skin breakages, swelling, blisters or discomfort. Report any changes to the patient's feet to the senior nurse, and document care given.

Facial shaving

Facial shaving is an important part of the over all appearance and well being of the patient (excluding some Sikh males). If a man usually shaves everyday, being unshaven can feel uncomfortable and can look as if the patient is uncared for. Most patients will be able to shave themselves, sometimes encouragement may be required if the patient has lost interest in their appearance. Helping to

promote the patient's independence can be vital in aiding their recovery. Some men may be anxious if someone else is going to shave them. To help relieve their anxiety, it is important to reassure them that you are competent at performing the task. If female patients wish to shave, healthcare assistants should ensure privacy and confidentiality in order to maintain the patient's dignity.

Using an electric shaver is an alternative to wet shaving. It is important to note that razors should never be shared between patients to avoid infection. It is important to be aware if a patient has a blood disorder or is receiving anticoagulant therapy as these patients should ideally use an electric shaver. If a patient is cut during the procedure apply pressure using a piece of gauze until the bleeding has stopped (Jevon and Jevon, 2001).

Equipment required for a wet shave
- Non-sterile gloves and disposable apron
- Bowl of warm water
- Towel
- Disposable wipes
- Mirror
- Razor (either disposable, or the patient's own)
- Shaving foam/gel
- Shaving brush
- After-shave or lotion.

Procedure
- Greet patient and explain procedure
- Wash hands and put on gloves and apron
- If possible sit the patient in an upright position
- Place a towel around the patient's shoulders and across the chest
- Place a mirror in front of the patient so they can see what you are doing
- It is important to examine the patient's face before commencing to observe for any skin irritations, cuts or rashes
- Wet the patient's face with warm water using a disposable wipe, this helps to soften the hairs and relax the facial muscles
- Apply the shaving foam/gel using the shaving brush, or massage onto the face using your gloved fingers until there is a lather. This helps moisten and soften the patient's skin
- Hold the razor in your dominant hand at a 45-degree angle and use the other hand to keep the surrounding skin taut
- Shave in the direction of the hair, never shave in the opposite direction of hair growth as this pulls the skin in the wrong direction, causing irritation and grazing of the skin

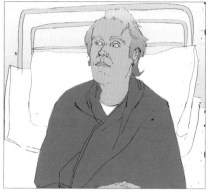

1. If possible sit the patient in an upright position.

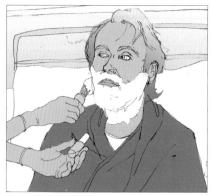

2. Apply the shaving foam/gel using the shaving brush, or massage onto the face using your gloved fingers until there is a lather.

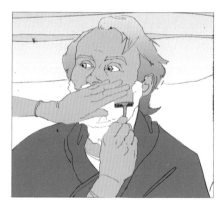

3. Shave in the direction of the hair.

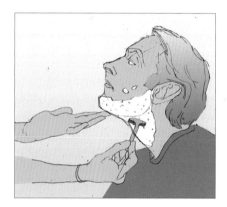

4. Start with the cheeks, followed by the neck, finishing with the chin and upper lip.

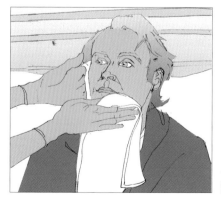

5. When shaving is complete wash the patient's face using a disposable wipe.

- Start with the cheeks, followed by the neck, finishing with the chin and upper lip. If possible ask the patient to position their face appropriately to aid the shaving procedure
- In-between shaving rinse the razor regularly in the bowl of warm water to remove the soap and hairs
- When shaving is complete wash the patient's face using a disposable wipe to remove any excess soap and hair
- Dry the face by gently patting it with a towel
- Apply after-shave or lotion if required
- If the razor is no longer sharp dispose of it in the sharps bin provided
- Ensure the patient is comfortable
- Dispose of your apron and gloves and wash and dry your hands
- Document care.

Cultural beliefs in relation to washing and dressing

Islam

Islam observes a strict segregation of the sexes so that many Asian women may be found resistant to uncovering the body or to physical contact and may react adversely to physical examination by male doctors or healthcare workers. Since Asian dress has religious significance, it is meant to cover all of the body including the legs. Some may be reluctant to wear Western type nightdresses, pyjamas or any style of hospital gown. Free flowing water is preferred so showers are often preferable to baths.

Sikhs

Sikh women prefer to be examined by female doctors and healthcare workers, and always have their legs and arms covered. They prefer showers to baths. Sikh men may not shave their beards. Hair is always kept clean and covered. A kanga is used to keep the hair in a bun on top of the head, a turban is then placed over the hair. Usually a Sikh man is reluctant to remove his turban.

Hindus

Hygiene can have important religious significance in Hinduism. Showers are preferable to baths, as Hindus like to wash in free flowing water. They also like to use mouthwashes after eating. Some Hindus may be distressed if the anal region is not washed with water or a damp tissue after a bowel action. The right hand is usually used for 'clean' tasks, the left for 'unclean' tasks. Hindu women may refuse to be examined or undress in front of males. They may also find open backed theatre gowns unsuitable, however they can wear closed nightdresses and pyjama bottoms. Many Hindu women and young girls wear markings on their forehead. This traditionally indicates that a women is married, however it can be worn as make-up. (Yonwin, 2000). Married women also wear wedding jewellery and removal should be avoided as this can cause distress.

Other cultures

The care of hair is important to Afro-Caribbean people. After washing the hair a conditioner or light oil may be required to prevent the hair from becoming too dry. Some women also like to wear scarves. Afro-Caribbean and many other African cultures use oils and moisturisers on their skin as taking care of themselves is seen as a sign of self-respect.

Privacy and dignity

The privacy and dignity of patients should be considered at all times. It is of the utmost importance when caring for patients' personal hygiene needs. Support should be given that encourages patients to do as much for themselves as possible to maintain their independence and physical ability. This also encourages patients with disabilities to make the most of their own potential and independence. Individuals have the right to be respected, be treated equally and not be discriminated against, be treated as an individual, be treated in a dignified way (DH, 2003).

Safeguarding the privacy of the patient means to be protected from danger and harm, be cared for in the way that meets their needs, have a choice, have access to information about themselves, and communicate using their preferred method of communication and language (Skills for Health, 2004).

The term body image is the picture we have of ourselves. It can be upsetting for patients to see a change in their body, as this alters the picture they usually have of themselves. It is important when caring for patient's with an altered body image to be supportive and give reassurance. Also allow the patient time to express their feelings. Conditions that may affect a patient's body image include:

- Scarring
- Loss of limb (amputation)
- Removal of breast (mastectomy)

- Skin conditions
- Weight loss
- Hair loss
- Opening of the bowel on to the abdomen (colostomy)
- Paralysis of a limb (hemiplegia) caused by a stroke
- Wounds or burns (Yonwin, 2000).

It is also important to give patients the choice to wear their own clothes. Clothes are worn for warmth, protection and for individual expression, also for different cultural and religious reasons. It is important to ensure that the patient's clothes are clean and changed as required. Some patients may need assistance with dressing and undressing and there are many different aids available to help individuals (Yonwin, 2000). Some patients may require different pieces of equipment to help with certain medical conditions they have (*Table 3*).

Conclusion

Providing patients with a high standard of personal hygiene care, whether in the hospital or community setting, is vital for their mental and physical wellbeing. The healthcare assistant's role is vital in ensuring that this is

Table 3. Equipment to help with certain conditions	
Category of patient aid	**Type of patient aid**
Sensory equipment	Hearing aids
	Spectacles
Artificial body part (prosthesis)	Artificial limb
	False eye
	False breast
	Toupee or wig
	Dentures
Specialist equipment	Surgical shoes
	Calipers
	Braces
	Collars
	Corsets
	Splints

achieved. For healthcare assistants to be able to provide this high standard of care they need to have a basic knowledge of the functions of the skin, be able to assess patients with different abilities, understand the principles of privacy and dignity, and have an insight into different cultures. Finally, they need to have good communication skills and understand the importance of accurate and clear documentation. Providing healthcare assistants with these skills and knowledge is fundamental if patients are going to receive a high standard of care. Understanding the theory and having the knowledge base is key before applying it to practice. When the skills are applied to practice it is important that the healthcare assistant is assessed as competent by an experienced practitioner before they are able to perform the care independently.

Ambrose M, Quinless F (2004) Fundamental procedures. In: *Nursing Procedures*. 4th ed. Lippincott, Williams and Wilkins, Philadelphia: 1-114

Ashurst A (2003) NVQ in Care — Maintaining client hygiene and appearance. *Nursing and Residential Care* **5**(3): 104–109

Baker F, Smith l, Stead L (1999c) Washing a patient's hair in bed. *Nursing Times* **95**(5): 20

DH (2003) *Essence of Care: Patient Focused Benchmarks for Healthcare Practitioners*. DH, London

Doughtery L, Lister S (2004) *The Royal Marsden Hospital Manual of Clinical Procedures*. Blackwell Publishing, Oxford

Jevon P, Jevon M (2001) Practical Procedure for Nurses: Facial shaving. *Nursing Times* **97**(11): 43–45

Nursing Times clinical skills update (2003a) Oral hygiene: Why it is important. *Nursing Times* **99**(1): 29

Nursing Times clinical skills update (2003b) Bedbaths: Why give bed baths? *Nursing Times* **99**(5): 29

Pegram A, Bloomfield J, Jones A (2007) Clinical skills: bed bathing and personal hygiene needs of patients. *British Journal of Nursing* **16**(6): 356–358

Rhind J, Greig (2002) *Riddles in Anatomy and Physiology Applied to Health Professionals*. Churchill Livingstone, Edinburgh

Skills for Health (2003) *Support individuals with their personal care needs. https://tools. skillsforhealth.org/competence/show?code=HSC218<file;??localhost/competence/show* (accessed 13 October 2008)

Waugh A and Grant A (2006) *Ross and Wilson Anatomy and Physiology in Health and Illness*. Churchill Livingstone Elsevier, Edinburgh

Yonwin H (2000) Self-Directed Learning -Enabling clients to maintain their personal hygiene and appearance. *Nursing and Residential Care* **2**(5): 243-247

CHAPTER 6

Pressure ulcer prevention

Menna Lloyd-Jones

It is estimated that around 412,000 individuals per annum will develop a pressure ulcer. The annual cost to the NHS is estimated to be between £1.4 and £2.1 billion, which represents 4% of the total NHS expenditure (Bennett et al, 2004). However, it is impossible to put a cost on the unnecessary pain and discomfort that a patient with pressure ulcers has to endure. Havard (2007) emphasises that patients with pressure ulcers had to stay in hospital longer and also had to be readmitted with pressure ulcer related conditions. Pressure ulcer prevention is therefore very important and could save patients months of unnecessary pain and suffering, apart from the millions of pounds that could be saved to the NHS .

A pressure ulcer is defined as an area of localised damage to the skin caused by pressure, shear, friction and/or a combination of these (European Pressure Ulcer Advisory Panel [EPUAP], 2003).

In order to prevent pressure ulcers it is important to understand the anatomy and function of the skin as well as understand the causes of pressure ulcers and factors that can predispose the patient to pressure ulcer.

The skin

The skin is the largest organ in the body. It covers an area of approximately $2m^2$, constitutes almost one sixth of the total body weight and receives around one third of the body's circulating blood volume (Flanagan, 1997). The skin forms a barrier between the body and the external environment; it has a slightly acid pH of around 5.5 and is made up of two main layers, the epidermis and the dermis. Lying beneath the dermis is the hypodermis or subcutaneous layer (Timmons, 2006).

The epidermis it the outermost layer of the skin. It is avascular — which means that it has no blood supply — and receives oxygen and all its nutrients by diffusion from the dermis. The epidermis is very thin with a thickness of only 0.1mm in all areas with the exception of the palm of the hands and the sole of the feet where extra thickness is needed to protect this area which is used for either walking or handling. The thickness here can be between 1and 2mm (Butcher and White, 2005).

The epidermis is made up of five cell layers:

- *Stratum corneum*: the horny layer made up of dead keratinocytes, which are being constantly shed and replaced (Collins et al, 2002)
- *Stratum lucidum*: the clear layer only present on areas of the body such as the palms of the hands and soles of feet, where thickness is required to offer some further protection
- *Stratum granulosum*: the granular layer made up of dead un-flattened granular cells
- *Stratum spinosum*: the prickle cell layer made up of living cells which are constantly replacing the layers above
- *Stratum germinativum*: the basal layer a single layer of living cells and together with the prickle layer above form the germinative layer. These layers are constantly producing new cells, which move upwards and are eventually shed at the horny layer (Flanagan, 1997).

Once damaged the epidermis repairs itself by a process called regeneration. This means that it replicates itself as the cells of the basal layer multiply and move in a leapfrog fashion from undamaged areas to replace damaged cells. Replacing cells in this fashion leaves no visible scar (Eisinger, 1985).

The dermis is firmly attached to the epidermis at the dermal-epidermal junction. The dermis provides nutrition and support to the epidermis and is predominately made up of fibrous proteins, collagen and elastin (connective tissue), which gives the skin its strength and elasticity (Flanagan, 1997).

The dermis is made up of 2 layers:

- *The papillary layer*: the uppermost layer of the dermis which contains capillary loops, nerve endings, hair follicles, sweat glands, sebaceous glands, temperature and touch receptors and fine lymph vessels
- *The reticular layer*: although there is no clear division between the two layers, the main difference is in the gradual increase in size of the collagen fibres and in the size of the blood vessels (Flanagan, 1997).

The dermis cannot regenerate and heals by the formation of granulation tissue (growth of new tissue). Scaring is dependent on the depth of the damage and length of time the wound takes to heal (Eisinger, 1985). The strength of repaired tissue is around 80% the strength of undamaged tissue, in the same way the blood supply is less and will not support dermal appendages such as hair follicles, sweat glands or sebaceous glands (Timmons, 2006).

Below the dermis lies the subcutaneous layer or hypodermis. The subcutaneous layer is made of adipose tissue, connective tissue and contains larger blood vessels. This function of the subcutaneous layer is to provide support to the dermis and the fat stored in the subcutaneous layer provides protection to the internal structures as well as providing insulation against the cold (Timmons, 2006).

Functions of the skin

The skin has five main functions: it protects, it helps to regulate body temperature, it registers external stimulation, it metabolises vitamin D and melanin, and it helps us to communicate with each other.

Protection
Intact skin acts as a waterproof barrier and protects the body from bacteria and viruses and any break in the skin can put the individual at risk of developing infection. The skin also protects against mechanical damage and trauma such as that caused by pressure shear and friction (Butcher and White, 2005).

Temperature control
The skin helps control body temperature by cooling the body through the secretion of sweat by the sweat glands.

Sensation
Nerve receptors in the skin are sensitive to pain, pressure, touch, vibration as well as hot and cold (Flanagan, 1997).

Production
Vitamin D production is stimulated by sunlight and melanin production gives us our pigmentation and protect against the harmful rays of the sun (Butcher and White, 2005).

Communication
Effects of skin damage can be seen by observing the skin, for example changes in skin colour, its texture and its temperature.

The effects of ageing on the skin

Ageing results in both visible and structural changes to the skin, including the overall thinning of the epidermis which is particularly noted after the age of 70 years and is more prevalent in women than in men. Although there is thinning of the epidermis there is no evidence to suggest that the protective function of the skin is jeopardised (Desai, 1997). However, there are suggestions that the skin can become more susceptible to damage from mechanical forces such as moisture, friction and trauma (Wounds UK, 2006).

During the ageing process there is a flattening out of the dermo-epidermal junction, which makes it more fragile and more susceptible to tearing and trauma (Desai, 1997). The paper-thin appearance of elderly skin can be attributed to an estimated 20% reduction in the thickness of the dermis. The thinning of the dermis also causes a reduction in the blood supply, nerve endings and collagen, which in turn leads to a decrease in sensation, temperature control, rigidity and moisture control (Wounds UK, 2006). Wrinkles and skin folds appear due to changes in the architecture of the collagen and the elastic fibres which loose some of their elasticity. As a result the skin becomes less stretchable, less resilient and more lax (Desai, 1997; Burr and Penzer, 2005). There is also a reduction in the number of sweat glands which leads to dryness of the skin. Dry skin can lead to splitting and cracking which exposes the skin to contamination from bacteria thus increasing the risk of infection (Wounds UK, 2006). Incontinence is a problem associated with old age and urine and faeces can change the pH of the skin from acid to alkaline thereby increasing the risk of further damage to the skin.

The aetiology of pressure ulcers

There are three main causes of pressure damage and these are pressure, shear and friction.

Pressure occurs when the skin and other tissues are squeezed together between bone and a hard surface. The squeezing of the tissues interrupts the blood supply to the area, leading to ischemia (localised deficiency of arterial blood) and tissue death (Wounds UK, 2006). It has to be noted that it is not just the amount of pressure which causes the damage, as time is also a factor. For example high pressure for a short period of time or low pressure for a longer period of time can both result in pressure damage (Morris, 2007).

Friction is the force generated when two surfaces move across one another and can cause superficial damage such as stripping of the epidermis (Desai, 1997; Dealy, 1997). Incorrect manual handling — where the patient is dragged up a bed — is a common cause of friction damage.

Shearing is the stretching of the skin where the skeleton moves down and the skin remains where it is causing stretching and distortion of the blood vessels. This in turn can cause similar damage to the skin as pressure (Morris, 2007). An example of shear is a patient sliding down a bed or chair.

There are also predisposing factors that combined with pressure, friction and shear can put the patient at higher risk of developing pressure ulcers. It would be impossible to list all potential factors, however NICE (2005) have listed the following as factors that increases an individual's potential to develop pressure ulcers:

Acute illness
Acutely ill patients are vulnerable to developing pressure ulcers due to conditions such as heart failure, shock, pain, low blood pressure and temperature change which occur, for example during and after anaesthesia.

Mobility status
It is well documented that reduced mobility or immobility is a key factor in the development of pressure ulcers (Dealey, 1997).

Sensory impairment
Neurological deficit, for example diabetes, stroke and multiple sclerosis, results in reduced sensation and as a consequence the patient is not aware of pain or discomfort which is the normal stimulus for movement to relieve pressure.

Level of consciousness
A reduced level of consciousness may diminish an individual's awareness of the need to relieve pressure. In the same way anaesthetised patients cannot reposition themselves.

Nutritional status
Malnutrition may increase an individual's risk of organ failure and serious illness. Very thin patients have very little padding to protect bony prominence, and obese patients may have difficulty moving themselves while their weight and size makes them difficult to be move and handled by others. Dehydration may reduce the elasticity of tissues and make it more vulnerable to pressure, shear and friction.

Previous pressure damage
Previous history of pressure damage puts individuals at a greater risk of developing further ulcers compared with patients who have not previously developed pressure ulcers.

Pain status
Pain makes a patient reluctant to move and may affect their appetite therefore a pain assessment should include, whenever the individual is experiencing

pain, the cause of pain, level of pain (using appropriate tool), location and management interventions.

Age

An extreme of age (less than 5 years of age and over 65 years). As people age their risk of developing conditions such as heart disease, neurological conditions and problems with their circulations increases their risk of developing pressure ulcers. Changes to the elasticity and thickness of the skin add to this risk. Neonates and very young children are also at a greater risk as their skin is still maturing and their head-to-body weight is disproportionate.

Continence status

Incontinence can change the pH of the skin from acid to alkaline and can change the normal flora of the skin as well as rapidly causing maceration of the skin (softening of tissue that has remained wet or damp for a long period of time). Interventions to contain and manage the continence problems may impair the function of pressure relieving support surface, for example pads or bedding.

Medication

Sedatives and hypnotics may make an individual excessively sleepy and thus reduce mobility. Analgesics may reduce normal stimulus to relieve pressure.

Preventing pressure ulcers

Preventing pressure ulcer development is important and NICE (2005) highlights the importance of adequate risk assessment alongside skin inspection. Morris (2007) states that the healthcare assistant is in an ideal position to identify the first signs of pressure ulcers by regularly inspecting the skin.

Skin inspection

The frequency of skin inspection is dependent on the condition of the individual (NICE 2005). For example if a patient's condition is deteriorating they may need to have their skin inspected and their position changed as often as every two hours. However as their condition improves the skin inspection can be as little as once a day (NICE, 2005).

The skin inspection should include assessment of the most vulnerable areas at risk of pressure damage which are the sacrum, the buttocks, hips, heels, elbows and shoulders. If the patient is nursed on their back, for example due to a spinal injury, then the back of the head is also an area that needs to be checked.

Signs of possible damage

Check for a reddened area which when pressed does not turn white (non-blanching erythema). Also look out for any blistering especially on the heels. Other signs include warmth, swelling or hardness especially on patients with darkly pigmented skin where it is not possible to identify blanching or non blanching erythema. (See *Table 1* for the blanching test). Any skin changes must be reported.

EPUAP (2003) has graded pressure ulcers from a Grade 1, unbroken skin, to a Grade 4, deep tissue damage, through to muscle and bone (see *Table 2*).

Skin care

Incontinence has been identified as a risk factor in pressure ulcer development. However washing vulnerable areas with soap and water can change the pH of the skin and lead to dry skin. To reduce the drying effects of using soap and water the skin should be washed with a non-soap cleanser or emollient soap substitute. The skin should then be dried using a patting motion and a barrier cream applied as appropriate (Dealey, 1997; Wounds UK, 2007). The practice of rubbing reddened areas is not recommended as this can lead to shear damage (Waterlow, 2005).

Table 1.	The blanching test
1	Apply light fingertip pressure to the area of discoloration for 10 seconds
2	Release the pressure. If the area is white and then returns to its original colour, it probably has an adequate blood supply. Observation should continue and preventative strategies should be employed
3	If, on release of pressure, the area remains the same colour as before pressure was applied, it is an indication of the beginning of pressure ulcer development and preventative strategies should be employed immediately
4	If there is an alteration in the skin colour (redness, purple or black), increased heat or swelling, it may imply underlying tissue breakdown. Frequency of assessment should be increased and preventative strategies should be employed (Morris, 2007)

Equipment and repositioning

NICE (2005) recommend that all patients with pressure ulcers should have 24 hour access to pressure relieving equipment, which implies all support surfaces including trolleys and theatre tables. However, they do not recommend the use of equipment such as water filled gloves, sheepskins and doughnut type devices for pressure relief.

Pressure relieving equipment includes mattresses and cushions. Mattresses can be pressure reducing or pressure relieving. Pressure reducing mattresses include foam or visco-elastic foam mattresses. These work by redistributing the pressure — that is they spread the weight of the patient over a larger surface area. Pressure relieving mattresses include alternating pressure or air mattresses and work, for example, by relieving pressure as the cells of the mattress inflate or deflate under the patient (Beldon, 2007a).

NICE (2005) recommends that all patients at risk of developing

---

Table 2. The EPUAP pressure ulcer grading

Grade 1
Non-blanchable erythema of intact skin. Discoloration of the skin with warmth, oedema, induration or hardness may also be used as indicators, particularly on individuals with darker skin.

Grade 2
Partial thickness skin loss involving epidermis, dermis or both. The ulcer is superficial and presents clinically as an abrasion or blister.

Grade 3
Full thickness skin loss involving damage to or necrosis of subcutaneous tissue that may extend down to but not through underlying fascia.

Grade 4
Extensive destruction, tissue necrosis or damage to muscle, bone or supporting structures with or without full thickness skin loss.

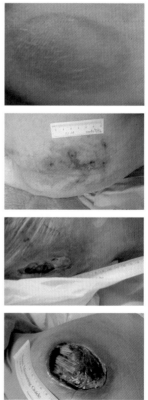

pressure ulcers should as a minimum be nursed on a pressure reducing mattress or cushion with pressure relieving properties, alongside planned repositioning schedules. The frequency of repositioning is determined by skin inspection and should be based on individual need. Patients that are able to reposition themselves must be encouraged to reposition as often as possible. Those in wheelchairs are encouraged to reposition themselves every 15 minutes. In order to minimize the risk of shear and friction damage when repositioning, consideration should be taken of good manual handing techniques (NICE, 2005).

Where possible patients should not be positioned directly onto pressure ulcers and all positional changes should be recorded on a repositioning or tuning chart (NICE, 2005).

Seating

Sitting for long periods of time has been recognized as a factor in the development of pressure ulcers, and NICE (2005) recommend that acutely ill patients should not be sat out of bed for more than two hours.

When seated the patient ideally should be sat with their feet flat on the floor, with their hips and knees at 90°. Where possible the thighs should be supported along the full length of the chair with two finger widths between the chair and the back of their knees and either side of their thighs (Beldon, 2007b). Poor sitting position can cause pain and discomfort as well as having an adverse effect on some of the internal organs and the patient's mental state (Simpson et al, 1997).

Nutrition

Nutrition has an important role in the prevention and treatment of pressure ulcers as a poor nutritional status can lead to a delay in wound healing and increase the patient's risk of developing an infection (Johnston, 2007). Maintaining a well balanced diet is important and every effort should be made to ensure that the patient is in a suitable position to eat their meals, have access to adapted cutlery, and if required ensure that food has been placed within reach and any wrapping removed (Dealey, 1997). Offer encouragement and praise. In order to increase the energy and protein content of the diet without increasing the volume consumed, where appropriate add cheese to mashed potatoes, for example, or replace semi-skimmed or skimmed milk with full fat milk (Johnston, 2007).

Meeting fluid requirements is also important and as a guide most people require 1500 ml of fluids daily, which equates to between eight and 10 cups or glasses. In order to assist with meeting daily fluid requirements ensure that the fluid is within reach, and where necessary offer a beaker or straw. High-fluid foods such as jelly, soup or fruit are also an option (Johnston, 2007).

Conclusion

Pressure ulcers can cause the patient a lot of unnecessary pain and discomfort and costs the NHS between £1.4 and £2.1 billion per annum. In order to prevent the development of pressure ulcers it is important to have an understanding of the anatomy and function of the skin, alongside the aetiology of pressure ulcers.

EPUAP and NICE have developed guidelines to aid in the management and treatment of pressure ulcers, and following theses guidelines can help to prevent the development of pressure ulcers and relieve the unnecessary suffering of patients.

Bennett G, Dealy C, Posnett J (2004) The cost of pressure ulcers in the UK. *Age Ageing* **33**(3): 230–5

Beldon P (2007a) Pressure ulcer prevention and management: Using mattresses and cushions. *Wounds Essential* **2**: 92–100

Beldon P (2007b) Sitting safely to prevent pressure damage. *Wounds Essential* **2**: 102–4

Burr S, Penzer R (2005) Promoting Skin Health. *Nursing Standard* **19**(36): 57–65

Butcher M, White R (2005) In: White R ed. *Skin Care in Wound Management: Assessment and Treatment*. Wounds UK. Aberdeen

Dealy C (1997) *Managing Pressure Sore Prevention*. Quay Books, London

Defloor T, Clark M, Pressure Ulcer Classification Self-Assessment. www.epuap.org/puclas/indexhtml. Accessed February 2007

Desai H (1997) Ageing and wounds part 2, healing in old age. *J Wound Care* **6**(5): 237–9

European Pressure Ulcer Advisory Panel. (2003) Pressure Ulcer Prevention Guidelines. www.eupap.org.uk

Eisinger M (1985) Regeneration of epidermis by cells grown in tissue culture. *J Am Acad Dermatol* **12**: 402–48

Flanagan M (1997) *Wound Management*. Churchill Livingstone, London

Havard D (2007) A snapshot of England's. *Wounds UK* **3**(2): 13–20

Johnston E (2007) The role of nutrition. *Wound Essentials* **2**: 10–20

Morris C (2007) Pressure ulcers part 1:aetiology and identification. *British Journal of Healthcare Assistants* **1**(2): 81–2

Simpson A, Bowers K, Weir-Hughes D (1997) *Pressure Sore Prevention*. Whurr, Tyne & Wear

The National Institute for Clinical Excellence (2005) *The management of pressure ulcers in primary and secondary care. A clinical guideline.* Royal Collage of Nursing, London

Timmons J (2006) Skin Function and Healing. *Wound Essentials* **1:** 8–17

Waterlow J (2005). Pressure Ulcer Prevention Manual. www.judy-waterlow.co.uk

Wounds UK (2006) *Best Practice Statement: Care of the Older Person's Skin.* Wounds UK, Aberdeen

CHAPTER 7

Principles of wound healing and management

Menna Lloyd-Jones

Wound care has developed rapidly over the past 20 years to become a complex and dynamic speciality. All healthcare practitioners involved with wound care should as a minimum have a basic understanding of the principles of wound care which are based on best practice, research-based evidence and expert consensus.

The physiology of wound healing

In order to be able to care for patients with wounds it is important to understand the normal process of wound healing (Dealy, 1999).

Wound healing can be defined as the physiology by which the body replaces and restores function to damaged tissue (Tortora and Grabowski, 1996). Wounds will heal in one of three different ways:

- Primary intention
- Secondary intention
- Delayed primary intention.

Primary intention (or first intention), the edges of the wound are brought together by sutures, paper strips or glue. Within 24–48 hours the epidermis (uppermost layer of the skin) will have sealed the surface of the skin, although healing will continue below this surface (Collins et al, 2002).

Secondary intention occurs when the edges of the wound cannot be brought together or where there is tissue loss and the wound is left to heal. Pressure ulcers and leg ulcers are examples of wounds that heal by secondary intention.

Delayed primary intention occurs when the wound edges are not brought together for the first few days following surgery. The patient may the be taken back to theatre to have the wound aligned and sutured, etc. This method of closure is used if for example a wound is infected or contaminated (Collins et al, 2002).

Wound healing is a complicated chain of events which is triggered by damage to tissue. The process can be divided into four overlapping stages (Young, 2004).

Inflammation

This can last 0–3 days. The aim of this stage is to reduce and arrest the blood loss and to facilitate the arrival of the necessary agents to start the healing process. Damage to tissue and blood vessels initiate the release of agents which cause the end of the damaged blood vessels to constrict (vasoconstriction) in order to reduce blood flow. At the same time platelets are attracted to the site of injury. The platelets combine with collagen in the walls of the damaged blood vessels to form a plug (Timmons, 2006). Vasoconstriction is followed by vasodilatation and increased permeability of the blood vessels which allows movement of fluids from the blood vessel into the tissue (Dealy, 1999). The inflammatory stage is characterised by:

- Redness — due to the increase in blood flow
- Heat — increase in blood flow causes an increase in local temperature
- Swelling — due to movement of fluid into the tissues
- Pain — due to increase in pressure from the extra fluid (Shipperely and Martin, 2002; Timmons, 2006).

Destruction

Can last between 1–6 days. During this stage of healing neutrophils and macrophages are responsible for the cleaning up process (which is called phagocytosis) where white blood cells engulf or ingesting bacteria, dead cells and/or foreign matter (Young, 2004).

Proliferation

Can last between 3–24 days. During this stage of healing the macrophages and fibroblasts start to rebuild damaged tissue. Macrophages produce substances which are responsible for stimulating the growth of new blood vessels (angiogenesis) and fibroblasts multiply and form a scaffold of collagen fibres into which new cells and blood vessels can travel (Young, 2004; Shipperely and Martin, 2002).

Maturation

This is the final stage of healing and can take up to between 21 days to 2 years. During this stage of healing the epithelial tissue moves from the wound edges across the wound bed, meeting to form a final cover of epithelial tissue. The provision of a moist wound environment aids this stage of healing as the epithelial cells can move across a moist environment quicker than having to burrow underneath a dry scab (Young, 2004; Shipperley and Martin, 2002).

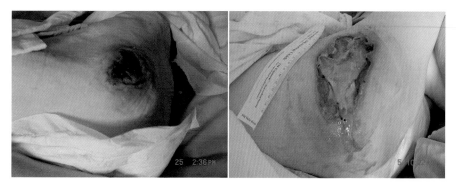

Figure 1. Inflammation.   Figure 2. Destruction.

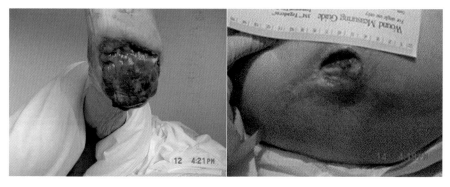

Figure 3. Proliferation.   Figure 4. Maturation.

Pain and wound care

Pain is something that is unique to each individual and includes both psychological and physiological factors (Lloyd Jones, 2004). Constant pain can have an adverse response on both wound healing and on quality of life. Collier and Hollinworth (2000) state that patients are more likely to experience wound pain during dressing change.

Definition

Pain, according to the International Association for the Study of Pain (IASP) (1994) is defined as:

> '...an unpleasant sensory and emotional experience associated with actual or potential tissue damage'.
>
> *IASP (1994)*

It also has to be recognised that pain is what the patient says it is (McCaffery, 1983). The experience of the practitioner undertaking the wound care procedure can, according to Douglas and Way (2006), have either a positive or negative influence on the patients and their pain. This is an important factor to consider when undertaking wound care procedures.

Mechanisms of pain

Wound pain is complex and predominately serves to protect from further trauma and to aid healing (Coulling, 2007).

As a rule, wound pain is usually classified as acute or chronic pain. The function of acute pain is to initiate a protective reaction and is felt instantly. It is easily localised and often described as a sharp or prickly pain which usually subsides with healing (Douglas and Way, 2006). Chronic pain on the other hand is of slower onset and is usually described as a burning or throbbing pain which continues even after healing is complete (Principles for Best Practice, 2004).

Causes of wound pain

In order to prevent or manage wound pain it is important to have a clear understanding of the causes of wound pain. Causes of pain can be described as follows:

- *Operative pain*: occurs as a result of interventions such as sharp or surgical debridement where dead devitalised tissue is removed with scissors or a scalpel. This is referred to as 'operative pain' and the procedure should only be performed by a clinician with specialist skills

- *Procedural pain*: occurs as a result of the actual wound care procedures which includes dressing removal, wound cleansing and reapplication of the dressing

- *Incident pain*: is movement related and occurs during day-to-day activities such as moving the patient, when the patient themselves cough, or if there is movement and/or slippage of the dressing

- *Background pain*: is felt at rest when no wound care procedure is being undertaken. The underlying pain is probably due to the cause of the wound itself and local wound factors such as a poor blood supply, infection, excoriation, maceration and patient related factors such as diabetes, rheumatoid arthritis, and peripheral vascular disease. Pain can also be due to conditions such as osteoarthritis and cancers which are not wound related. Background pain is a continuous pain and likened to toothache

- *Psychosocial/environment*: psychosocial/environmental factors include age, gender, previous experience of wound pain, culture, and environment, all of which can influence the patient's pain experience (Principles of Best Practice 2004).

Pain management

Pain assessment should be the role of the registered nurse, however the healthcare assistant has a role in preparing the environment and the patient before the procedure as well as observing the patient during the wound care procedure.

Where possible a quiet room should be selected where there is no distraction. The windows should be closed, and any fans and mobile phones should be switched off. All equipment required such as dressings should be at hand and any cleansing solution should be at the right temperature.

If the procedure is to be carried out by a healthcare assistant then the procedure should be explained to the patient; taking time to discuss the procedure with the patient may allay some of their fears and anxiety. However if you are unsure of the answers refer the question to a registered nurse. Do not rush the patient, especially those patients suffering from dementia or confusion, as the need for dressing changes may not be clearly understood and rushing them can cause anxiety. If pain relief is required before the procedure ensure that the patient has taken their medication at least 30 to 45 minutes before you begin the procedure.

In order to prevent any discomfort to the patient assess the need for assistance to position the patient. Comfort and talk to the patient throughout the procedure; explain what is happening, stopping the procedure if the patient requires time out. Leave the wound exposed for as little as possible and avoid unnecessary stimulation of the wound as the slightest touch may cause pain (Briggs and Torra i Bou, 2002). If you are applying or removing dressings you should be familiar with the manufacturers' instructions. Before leaving the patient ensure that the dressing applied is comfortable and not causing any pain or discomfort and that the patient knows how to contact a member of the healthcare team if they develop pain and discomfort (Principles of Best Practice, 2004).

Wound cleansing

Wound cleansing has been identified as a source of wound pain, and as wound cleansing is not necessary in all circumstances it is important to follow the plan of care and carry it out only if specified. If there is a need to remove dressing residue, clean the surrounding skin or remove debris. Irrigation with warm cleansing solution is the preferred method of wound cleansing (Hollinworth and White, 2006). However, there is risk of splash back from this method and reasonable precautions should be taken to avoid contamination from splash back (Oliver, 1997). If irrigation is not an option then the wound should be cleansed with the recommended warm solution using non-woven gauze.

Wound cleansing solutions

Dealy (1999) considers saline 0.9% to be the only completely safe cleansing agent, however tap water is becoming more popular especially for the cleansing of leg ulcers. The concerns with regards to contamination from non-sterile water supplies appear to be unfounded. Nevertheless, it is recommended that tap water is allowed to run for a few minutes before wound cleansing (Flanagan, 1997).

Bathing and showering is also becoming increasingly popular, in particular for leg ulcers and sacral or perianal wounds, and are not only very refreshing for the patient but can also assists with the removal of the old dressings. However, it is not advisable to let the patient soak the wounds for long periods of time as open wounds have a tendency to absorb water which can result in an increase in the amount of exudate in the following few days (Flanagan, 1997; Pudner, 1997).

Temperature of cleansing solutions

As the temperature of the wound directly affects wound healing (Laurence, 1996) it is important that any cleansing solution used should be warmed to body temperature before use. Following cleansing it can take a wound as long as 40 minutes to regain its original temperature and up to three hours for wound healing activities to return to normal (Myers, 1982).

Dressings

Up until the nineteenth century dressings applied to wounds could be anything from spider's webs to rags. However, with the industrial revolution and the development of the textile industry came the manufacture of vast amounts of cheap material such as gauze and lint which could be used as dressings. At the end of the nineteenth century a surgeon called Gamgee started to use cotton wool as a surgical dressing and later combined it with fine open-weave gauze to form an absorbent dressing called Gamgee which incidentally is still in use to this day (Flanagan, 1997). The development of modern dressings as we know them today was still a long way off and their development was influence by the work of George Winter, who in 1962 published his work on moist wound healing. In 1973 stomahesive wafers, which were developed to protect the skin surrounding stomas, became available and were later produced as dressings which became known as hydrocolloid dressings (Flanagan, 1997). Today there are hundreds of different dressings, and although Gamgee is still available in the UK it is rarely used as a primary dressing (a dressing which is applied directly on to the wound bed).

With so many dressings available on the market dressing selection has become a complex process. One of the principal reasons for applying a dressing is to provide healing that is rapid and cosmetically acceptable. Dressings are also used to manage exudate and prevent infection, as well as reducing pain whilst causing minimal distress to the patient. Therefore dressing selection should always begin with a holistic assessment of the patient and a thorough assessment of the wound should be undertaken by a healthcare professional with the appropriate knowledge and competency in wound care (Morris, 2006).

Types of dressing

It is beyond the remit of this chapter to discuss all the different dressing types available and therefore only some of the most frequently used dressings are described below.

Alginate dressings are derived from seaweed and contain calcium or sodium alginate. Alginate dressings interact with the wound forming a hydrophilic gel on contact with exudate or blood and should therefore not be used on dry wounds. Alginates can be used with infected or sloughy wounds as well as to pack cavity wounds. The dressings come as flat dressings, ribbon and rope as well as some which are extra absorbent. They are suitable for use on moderate to heavy exuding wounds, e.g. pressure ulcers, leg ulcers or fungating wounds. They are useful for filling cavity wounds but care should be taken not to over-pack the wound They are also used with wounds that bleed as they have haemostatic properties. As the dressing is meant to mop up exudate it should not be moistened before use as this will affect the gelling process and may affect the capacity to absorb exudate. Depending on level of exudate and alginate dressing can be left in place for approximately five days.

Hydrocolloid dressings are a development from stoma care. They consist of a hydrocolloid base made from cellulose, gelatines and pectins, with a polyurethane film or foam backing. Hydrocolloids are interactive in contact with wound exudate and provide a viral barrier. They are indicated for wounds with a low to moderate exudate, e.g. pressure ulcers and leg ulcers. They are used to aid with the removal of necrotic (dead tissue) and sloughy wounds. However, hydrocolloid dressing may produce a slight malodour, which is normally more apparent on removal. Warming the dressing for three to five minutes before and after application can aid the application and adherence of the dressing. Allow at least a 2cm overlap around the wound edge. To remove, gently peel it off ensuring that underlying skin is not stripped.

Foam dressings are made from polyurethane foam or silicone. They are available as a flat dressing or cavity wound dressings. They are indicated for use with the management of low to heavily exuding wounds, e.g. leg ulcers, pressure ulcers, burns and donor sites. Cavity wound dressings can be used for filling large cavity wounds such as dehisced surgical wounds and pressure ulcers. Foam absorbs exudate and allows fluid to evaporate out of the dressing and therefore should not be covered with another dressing as this will inhibit the absorbency of the dressing. Foam dressings are not suitable for dry superficial wounds or those with a scab or dry necrotic eschar unless they are to be used for protection. Foam has no pressure relieving properties and should not be used in the prevention of pressure ulcers.

Film dressings are thin, vapour-permeable, hypoallergenic, adhesive coated film dressings which are permeable to both water vapour and oxygen, but are impermeable to micro-organisms. They provide a moist environment by reducing water vapour loss from the wound site. They are indicated for shallow wounds such as donor sites, minor burns, grazes and surgical incisions. They can be used to prevent the development of pressure ulcers by reducing friction and can also be used to cover blisters and grade I (non-blanching erythema) pressure ulcers. They are also used as a secondary dressing over a hydrogel dressing or alginate. However as previously mentioned they should not be used to hold a foam dressing in place. When removing a film dressing, lift the edge and stretch the dressing horizontally away from the wound.

Hydrogel dressings have a high water content and are indicated for use on dry necrotic and sloughy wounds. Hydrogels can also promote pain relief by keeping exposed nerve endings moist. In general hydrogels will need a secondary dressing therefore try and use a dressing that will not absorb the gel such as a film dressing or a non-adherent dressing such as a Telfa. If this is not practical, a foam dressing can be used. However hydrogels should not be used with an alginate, hydrofibre or hydrocolloid dressings and it is not advisable to use a hydrogel on heavily exuding wounds as the hydrogel will only add to the high level of exudate.

Hydrofibre dressings are highly absorbent non-woven dressings or ribbon dressings composed entirely of hydrocolloid fibres. On contact with exudate they convert from a dry dressing to a soft gel. They are indicated for use on moderately exuding wounds, pressure ulcers, leg ulcers, burns, surgical wounds and wounds prone to bleeding. They can be used on infected or fungating wounds and can be used to lightly pack cavity wounds, sinuses or fistulas. Like alginates, hydrofibres should not be used on dry wounds or wounds with very low exudate. They should be placed dry, leaving an overlap of at least 1cm over the wound edges and require a secondary dressing. On removal if the dressing is dry irrigating with warm sterile saline or water may be required to aid removal and then the findings should be reported so that the dressing selection can be reviewed before a new dressing is reapplied.

There are several different examples of the dressing types described above in daily use. Have a look at the dressings in your area and see if you can find an example of each category mentioned above. If you want to learn more about these dressings have a look at the information provided in the box with the dressing and every time you use a dressing consider what type of dressing it is and its intended use. And just a last word on dressings, do not make dressing sandwiches! You should only require a maximum of two dressings on a wound; if you have more than two then you may need to reconsider or seek advice.

When you undertake any wound care procedure remember to follow your local protocols for wound care and infection control.

Conclusion

The aim of this chapter was to give the reader an insight into the basics of wound care. It is in no way a complete guide to wound care and should serve only to enable the reader to deliver basic wound care under the instructions of healthcare professionals with the skills, knowledge and competencies to prescribe clinically effective wound care. Local protocols should always be followed.

Beldon P (2004) Is wound healing delayed in older patients? *Nursing in Practice* **Sept/Oct:** 73–6

Collins F, Hampton S, White R (2002) *A-Z dictionary of wound care.* Quay Books, London

Collier M, Hollinworth H (2000) Pain and tissue trauma during dressing change. *Nursing Standard* **14**(40): 71–3

Coulling S (2007) Fundamentals of pain management in wound care. *British Journal of nursing* **16**(11 suppl): S4–S12

Dealy C (1999) *The Care of Chronic Wounds.* Blackwell Science, London

Douglas V, Way L (2006) The assessment of wound pain: a review. *Practice Nursing* **17**(11): 532–42

Flanagan M (1997) *Managing wounds, Wound Management.* Churchill Livingstone, London

Flanagan M (1999) *The physiology of wound healing. in Wound management theory and practice.* NT books, Friary press, London

International Association for the Study of Pain Task Force on Taxonomy (1994) Classification of Chronic Pain. 2nd edn. Merskey H, Bogduk N eds IASP press, Seatle: 209–14

Lawrence JC, Harding KG, Moore DJ (1996) The use of antiseptics in wound care (three critiques). *Journal of Wound Care* **5**(1): 44–7

Lloyd Jones M (2004) Minimising pain at dressing changes. *Nursing Standard* **18**(24): 65–70

McCaffery M (1983) *Nursing a patient in pain.* Harper Row, London

Morris C (2006) Wound management and dressing selection. *Wounds Essential* **1**: 178–83

Myers JA (1982) Modern plastic surgical dressings. *Health Society Service Journal* **4**: 336–7

Oliver L (1997) Wound Cleansing. *Nursing Standard* **11**(20): 47–51

Principles of Best Practice (2004) *Minimising pain at wound dressing-related procedures.* A Consensus document. MEP Ltd, London

Pudner R (1997) Wound cleansing. *Journal of Community Nursing* **11**(7): 30–6

Shipperley T, Martin C (2002) The physiology of wound healing: an emergency response. *NT plus, wound care* **98**: 8

Timmons J (2006) Skin function and wound healing. *Wounds Essential* **1**: 8–17

Tortora GJ, Grabowski SR (1996) *Principles of Anatomy and Physiology.* Harper and Row Publications, New York

Young T (2004) The healing of amputation wounds. *Nursing Standard* **18**(45): 74–8

CHAPTER 8

Nutrition and oral hygiene

Angela Grainger

It is an essential part of any nurse's duty to ensure that patients' dietary needs are met:

> *'Hospital food is an essential part of patient care. Good food can encourage patients to eat well, aiding their recovery from surgery or illness. Patients should receive food that is safe, of good quality, nutritious, well presented and served at a time convenient to them.'*
>
> DH (2007a)

Without the necessary fuel and building materials the human body can neither repair, grow, heal itself, maintain itself, nor carry out any mental or physical activity whatsoever. Fuel and building materials all have to be provided by the input of food and water into the body. This input of food and water is what we mean by *nutrition*. The body's internal processing of this food and water so that it can be absorbed for delivery to the tissue which needs it is referred to as *digestion*. This is achieved by the processes of digestion. The word *diet* refers to the range and quantity of food and drink which a particular person accepts, or is able to consume, over a period of time. A diet, or a single foodstuff, which provides a good healthy intake is said to be *nutritious*. Inside the human body, nutrition triggers, fuels, and/or becomes part of many different chemical reactions. These processes are referred to as *metabolism*.

It is especially important for healthcare assistants to appreciate that when a person is combating an illness or recovering from injury they need to ensure that the diet provided contains a range and quantity of components, usually over-and-above the patient's normal intake level, to fuel this extra metabolism. In a nursing context, *diet* is not normally a reference to the latest social trends in eating patterns, it refers to the regime of foodstuffs that the patient must consume in order to help recovery.

> *'Patients who receive good nutrition may have shorter hospital stays, fewer post-operative complications and less need for drugs and other interventions.'*
>
> DH (2007b).

Components of nutrition

The essential foodstuffs for the human body are proteins, carbohydrates, fats, vitamins, and trace elements (often contained in minerals). Water is also absolutely essential in our diet. The body also needs an input of fibre. Fibre is an important aid to digestion but is not actually absorbed by the body and so does not enter any of our cells. Some people do not regard pure water as falling within the definition of food, and some food scientists also exclude fibre-only products from the strict definition of food. It must be remembered, though, that regular intakes of water are essential to keep us alive, and fibre is important to have a healthy digestive process.

Proteins

Proteins can be thought of as the substances which build or repair the tissues which make up our body (examples of human tissue are skin, bone, muscle, hair, blood vessels, and even blood itself). The main examples of foods which contain high levels of protein are meat, fish, cheese, milk and eggs. Some vegetables also have quite a high protein content, especially peas and beans. Nuts are another good source. Proteins are especially important for maintaining, building, and repairing muscle.

Carbohydrates

Carbohydrates are a type of substance found in all plants and animals, and are essential to our structure and functioning. Even our DNA is made partly from carbohydrates. As nutritional intake carbohydrates are the main fuel on which our body runs. There are many types of carbohydrates, including sugars and starches. They all have a similar, but very complex, chemical structure. The chemical structure of each type dictates what our body will do with it when eaten. For this reason, nutritionists tend to divide carbohydrates into saccharide categories. The two categories you should be aware of are the monosaccharides, and the disaccharides. The monosaccharides (meaning single sugars) include glucose (also called dextrose) and fructose (the sugar contained in fruit). Disaccharides (double sugars) include lactose (a type of sugar found in milk) and maltose (malt sugar). Table sugar, the sort we might add to tea or coffee, is technically called sucrose. It is a disaccharide (double sugar) consisting of glucose and fructose combined.

Food which is high in carbohydrates is often called high-energy food because some of the carbohydrate we eat will be used by our body as fuel. Some of it, though, will be converted into a different form called glycogen, and stored in our body for possible later use. Typical foodstuffs high in carbohydrates include most confectionary such as chocolate, sweets, cake, and biscuits. Pastry and bread are also major sources. Starchy foods such as potatoes and breakfast cereals are major sources too, and we must not forget about the carbohydrate content of sweet drinks and alcoholic drinks.

Fats

Fats are found in most animal flesh and in some vegetables, and even in some fruits. They are oily or greasy substances and are sometimes referred to on food labels as animal oils or vegetable oil. Nearly all the cells of our body naturally contain some fat, but its main function in our diet is to provide energy (fuel). Fat produces about twice as much body fuel as the same amount of carbohydrate will do, but the body needs more time to convert the fat to energy than it takes to convert carbohydrate to energy. Consequently, there is often a lot of fat from our food which our body never gets around to using and this is what leads to an obese appearance and the dangerous deposits of fat which can collect in (and risk blocking) our blood vessels. Foods high in fat are fatty meat, oily fish, nuts, and some seeds. Cheese, cooking oil, chocolate, confectionery and milk products can also contain high levels of fat.

Fats in mammal meat and some poultry (known as saturated fats) also contain cholesterol. Fats from vegetable sources and from fish oil (unsaturated fats) do not. A certain amount of cholesterol is needed by the cells in our body and also to make bile, but our liver can actually make cholesterol for us, so a diet rich in animal fats may give us too much cholesterol and this can do permanent damage to our blood vessels and dangerously restrict the circulation of blood. Butter, egg yolk, red meat, and shrimps contain relatively high levels of cholesterol. On the good-news side, the oil in salmon, mackerel, and tuna apparently helps to counteract the effect of cholesterol.

Vitamins

Vitamins are naturally-occurring chemicals present in some foods, and without a periodic intake of these we suffer ill-health. They are only needed in fairly small amounts. The vitamins are sometimes referred to by chemical names (such as thiamine), but more usually by a classification which uses letters (such as vitamin B, or vitamin B_1). Meat, fish, eggs, milk, fruit, and vegetables, for instance, all contain vitamins. Some foods contain only one or two vitamins, others contain several. Vitamins A, B (which is actually a group of related vitamins), C, D, and K are all essential. A varied and well balanced diet which includes fresh fruit and vegetables can provide all the vitamins needed, but tablets can be purchased fairly cheaply to supplement the diet of those for whom this is necessary.

Trace elements

Trace elements are naturally occurring substances, or combinations of substances (called minerals), found in various plants, animals or rocks. There are only a few of them which we need for our health, and the quantities we need are tiny. The most important examples are iron (present, for example, in meat, eggs, and green vegetables) and calcium (found, for example, in milk, eggs, and cheese). As with vitamins, a varied and well balanced diet which includes fresh fruit and vegetables can provide all the trace elements we need. Excess of some of some trace elements can be toxic.

The vast majority of foods, whether natural or processed, contain a mixture of some or all of the main nutritional substances described above. Virtually all will also contain some water, though it may not be obvious to either your eyes or to your taste buds. Cooking can substantially affect the nutritional content and value of foods, as can manufacturing processes such as rendering, re-forming, skinning, peeling, skimming, filleting, dehydrating, re-hydrating, re-constituting, blending, colouring, freezing, pre-cooking, adding water, canning, extending shelf-life, and so on. Generally, any type of cooking is likely to remove or reduce vitamin content, and will often add fat and/or water, but sometimes it can have the opposite effect. It depends on the precise food and the precise method. The same is true of processing.

Long-term storage can reduce the nutritional value of some foods. Food packagers now have to put the nutritional details on their labelling. This is of no help when it comes to fresh produce which we purchase unpackaged, of course, but plenty of books are available to help those who need to know and this includes healthcare assistants who might be working in certain community settings, including the patient's own home, and who might be expected to cook and prepare simple meals. In the hospital environment professional dieticians will have thoroughly assessed all the patients' food for nutritional content taking storage, cooking, and processing into account.

Appropriate nutrition

How much do we actually need to eat and drink? The answer to this depends on what body we have, and what we are calling upon it to do. The energy value of foods is measured and stated in terms of calories, or kilojoules. Every protein, carbohydrate and fat provides calories. Vitamins, trace elements and water do not. Fibre and cellulose do not provide any calorific content either since all it they do is pass straight through our body without being absorbed.

The more we are calling on our body to do, the more calories we need to give it. If we need to heat our body more (if we live in a cold climate, or because we are temporarily outdoors in very cold weather) it takes more calories to do this. A lumberjack or a sportsperson or a soldier is likely to need more calories than someone working in a call-centre.

A baby is doing more growing than an adult is and this calls for extra calories.

Someone who works standing up and walking about needs more calories than would be needed to do the same job entirely from a sitting position.

In general, adult males have larger bones and larger internal organs than adult females. A larger, heavier, skeleton needs more fuel and more tissue. That is why, as a general rule, men need more calories than women doing the same activity in a similar situation. An active teenager who is also still growing will need more calories than a fully grown adult who is elderly and not very mobile. Adolescents (particularly boys) undergoing a growth spurt may temporarily need more food than other teenagers.

Note also that the brain is a very fuel-hungry organ, and that when it is working hard for long periods of time, it can use a surprising amount of calories, and when both the body and brain are hard at work the nutritional replacement needed can be higher than you might expect.

It will be obvious from these examples that recommended calorie intake is only a general guide. The caloric intake currently recommended by the UK government is 2000 kcals per day for women, and 2500 kcals per day for men.

We also need to think about what proportion of our food should be protein, carbohydrate, or fat. Again, we can only generalise unless we are dealing with a specific individual person's needs. Our intake of fat should be low. We only need to eat enough fat to support and insulate certain internal organs, plus a small reserve for energy which is not immediately demanded. We need enough carbohydrate to fuel our current or imminent activity, and we need enough protein to build, repair, and maintain the structures of our body, particularly our muscles.

Water intake also depends on individual circumstances, but no adult should be having less than 2 litres of water per day. Hot weather, extreme physical exertion, and certain types of diet will all cause a person to need more water. Every part of the human body needs water, and when the body's water content becomes too low for proper functioning, cells (the various types of microscopically tiny living structures of which every one of our organs and tissues are composed) begin to dry out. This means that the person has become dehydrated, and if this problem is allowed to deteriorate and is not corrected death will eventually occur. Dehydration, even when it is only just beginning and is not an actual threat to health at that stage, is indicated by a feeling of thirst. Eventually the skin seems to look parched and dry and loses its elasticity.

Levels of vitamins and minerals are not a problem for most people in wealthy countries, but might not be sufficient at times of specially high demand such as during pregnancy. In developing countries, vast numbers of people, even if they survive periodic famines, are generally under-supplied with all the nutritional components needed for good health.

People who are homeless, or who are severely mentally ill, or who are very frail but living alone, or those who have very little money, are unlikely to be on a good quality, healthy diet which is sufficient in quantity and well-balanced in all the necessary components. A large proportion of people admitted to hospital or to residential care homes or nursing homes come directly from these circumstances and so may need therapeutic medically-recommended and monitored diets for at least a time. Do not assume, though, that people who are almost starved will be ravenously hungry and will pounce on any food offered. After a several weeks with very little or no food the digestive system has to be weaned gently back onto proper amounts of food, taking care not to overload a digestive system which has become very slow and sluggish through having had little to do for quite some time.

Special diets

Special diets are needed for people with certain medical conditions. People with diabetes mellitus have to have very close attention paid to the quantity of sugars they can ingest otherwise their blood glucose level becomes too high (hyperglycaemia). This can lead to cardiovascular complications such as stroke, heart attack, or to poor blood supply to the lower limbs so that ulcers occur. If a diabetic takes, or has too much of, the medication prescribed to help lower blood glucose levels but does not take-in a sufficient diet to work with this medication then too low a blood sugar can result (hypoglycaemia), and the patient will become pale, sweaty, and be generally confused and agitated. If either hyperglycaemia or hypoglycaemia remain uncorrected the patient will go unconscious and death can occur. Another example of special diet is a person with coeliac disease, who has to avoid foods containing the protein gluten found in wheat products.

Some patients might have to avoid certain foods or drinks whilst taking medication. This is to ensure that the efficacy of the medicine is not undermined in the treatment of the patient, and also so that no unwanted complications occur such as vomiting. This is why all medicinal products dispensed by pharmacists contain the manufacturer's information leaflet which states what the drug is, what it is for, the dosage, and any substances that you should not use when taking the product. The leaflet also states the side effects that might occur with the product and that a doctor must be consulted should these occur. Anyone taking medication, and certainly the healthcare professionals attending patients, must be aware of this information to ensure that medication is administered safely. Patients who have allergies must avoid any food substances that provoke an allergic reaction, for example, peanuts and shellfish. Most people who have to live with such restrictions have a good understanding of what is safe or unsafe for them in terms of food or drink so it is important that health professionals ask the patient about dietary needs as this is part of fundamental nursing care.

Diet and cultural care

Patients are individuals and they have a basic human right to have their need for certain food requirements on religious, cultural, or personal lifestyle preferences, to be respected. The nursing staff must do all they can to ensure that specially required foods are obtained; for example Muslim patients usually require halal meat. Where certain foods are to be avoided because they cause offence to patients these must not be offered, for example a patient who is Jewish may not accept pork. Vegetarians must not be offered meat products. Some faiths observe strict fasting during certain religious periods. Sometimes water is allowed to be ingested outside the permitted time for eating. The patient, or the patient's religious leader can advise the attending healthcare professionals on this.

More and more people now choose to adhere to dietary rules on ethical grounds or because of their own lifestyle choices. A vegan diet is a more extreme version of vegetarianism but some foods that vegetarians can accept such as cheese and eggs, a vegan cannot. If a patient has a dietary need that is difficult to meet within a normal hospital catering environment then a dietician should be consulted so that special arrangements can be made for the supply of the foodstuffs. Some hospitals allow the patient's family to bring in foodstuffs from home, whilst some, as part of their infection control policy, prefer this not to be done. Know what your employing organisation will allow, and if in doubt ask the registered nurse. If you are about to give food or drink to a patient and you are concerned about whether it is excluded by the patient's special dietary need you should discuss this with the patient or ask the registered nurse before the food is handed to the patient.

Some patients maintain themselves on a specific diet for slimming reasons and wish to stick to it whilst in hospital. Once again, this should be respected, although it might be best to advise the patient to mention this to the doctor treating them.

Malnutrition

Malnutrition literally means bad nutrition, and a person might be said to be malnourished as a result of it:

'Studies have shown that up to 40 percent of hospital patients are malnourished on admission.'

DH (2007b)

Malnutrition results from a period of time living on food which, overall, contains not enough or too much of any of the essential components — protein, carbohydrate, fat, vitamins, minerals, or water. Do not assume that someone suffering from malnutrition will be thin and starving. A malnourished person might be thin, of normal weight, or obese. It depends on the actual way in which their diet is wrong and therefore how the nutritional components interact with the body and the negative effects of this. For example, malnourishment occurs when a child is not getting fed enough protein and is consequently not growing properly, or in people who have too little calcium, with the consequence of thinning of the bone density.

Nutrition is a complicated science, yet most people manage the practicalities of it with reasonable success and without studying the complexities of it. When a person is receiving nursing care, whether in a hospital, or a community setting including the patient's own home, the professionals caring for them need to be more than normally aware of nutrition. You need to be alert to whether patients are eating and drinking enough. When people are ill, or when their ability to care for themselves is temporarily restricted or permanently impaired, their nutritional intake is more likely to be too little rather than too much. You need to have the practical skills to help people eat if they cannot manage properly alone. To be able to provide this very personal life-preserving and health-restoring service properly is very rewarding and satisfying for both the patient and the carer.

Before we look at the skills required in helping a patient to eat and drink we need to remind ourselves of the digestive process because how the nurse prepares a patient for eating and drink affects digestion.

Digestion

Normally all nutrition is taken in by mouth. The mouth is the opening to the digestive tract, which is the route which food takes through the body. The digestive tract runs from the mouth, down the oesophagus, into the stomach, and then through the intestines. The nutrients in our food and drink are extracted by various mechanisms along this route and are then absorbed for use. Waste, and any substance that cannot be absorbed, passes out of from body as faeces. Water and certain other by-products of metabolism is passed out of the body as urine.

Most of the metabolic processing of food is carried out by chemical reactions but some of the first stages are mechanical — in other words they

are physical actions performed by muscles and joints. These physical parts of nutrition and digestion necessitate important observations by nursing staff. First, there is chewing. This requires teeth (or dentures) to be present and in reasonably good condition. If your patient wears dentures these must be well-fitting and not cause any soreness or mouth ulcers. If the dentures are causing problems or are cracked then a dentist must see the patient so that new dentures are made. Saliva is produced in the mouth, and this helps to prepare food for swallowing. If a patient's lips appear very dry and cracked, this could be an indication of dehydration. It is a nursing responsibility to ensure that a patient's lips and mouth are kept in a good condition and this is why a section on oral hygiene is included later in this chapter. A patient who has a sore, cracked lip and whose mouth feels furred and unpleasant will not want to eat and drink, and so the vicious circle of the patient being malnourished and dehydrated, caused by poor oral hygiene, care continues.

The swallow reflex

For patients to be safe when eating they have to have a good 'swallow reflex'. The first phase of swallowing is a voluntary process of using your tongue to move some solid or liquid to the back of your mouth, but once this food or liquid is put there, swallowing it is a reflex action. A reflex action is an automatic action of nerves and muscles which a person cannot stop voluntarily. Anything which gets to that point *will* be swallowed, whether this is intended or not. The very important, indeed life-preserving, effect of the swallow reflex is that it prevents food from going down your airway into your lungs.

It is extremely important to know that the swallow reflex does not operate when a person is unconscious. This is why you must never give anything by mouth to someone who is unconscious. The swallow reflex can also be absent or not fully reliable in someone who is drowsy, drunk, intoxicated by narcotic substances, or who has certain neurological problems such as a stroke. Certain psychological disorders can also affect swallowing. If a patient's swallow reflex is in any doubt, a swallow reflex assessment will be undertaken by a speech and language therapist. Registered nurses are often taught this assessment skill so that should patients who need such an assessment be admitted during weekends or public holidays they are not deprived of food and drink for a long period before an assessment can be undertaken. This is a quality of care issue.

Once food or drink is in the digestive system, it is moved through the oesophagus (gullet), and later through the small and large intestine (also called the bowels) by an automatic process called peristalsis. Peristalsis can be visualised as waves of contraction so that a squeezing action is performed which moves the food content along the tube-shaped oesophagus, through

the stomach and along the intestines so that the digestive process continues. When a person has been immobile for some time peristalsis tends to be slower than usual and this can lead to constipation. In patients who have had abdominal surgery under a general anaesthetic peristalsis will temporarily be halted. These patients will be nil-by-mouth until the doctor or a registered nurse skilled in surgical nursing detects bowel sounds with a stethoscope. This indicates that peristalsis is resuming and the patient can commence to take small amounts of water. As this is tolerated, soup and a light diet is then given leading on to full diet.

Nausea and vomiting

Vomiting is peristalsis in reverse so that instead of food and drink moving down along the body, it is moved back through the digestive system and is ejected as vomit via the mouth. Vomiting is usually caused by something acting as an irritant, or is due to an obstruction. Nausea means the patient feels sick. Nausea might precede an episode of vomiting, or it might be something the patient is experiencing that occurs on its own. All episodes of nausea and/or vomiting should be reported to the registered nurse. If the patient is vomiting regularly then an intravenous infusion (a drip) might be inserted into the patient's arm to prevent dehydration and to correct any electrolyte imbalance in the blood. The healthcare assistant should observe the appearance and smell of vomit passed, and record the amount on a fluid balance chart. When a person is feeling nauseous it is best not to put food in front of them or to talk to them about eating or drinking. This can make the patient feel worse. When the patient is allowed to eat and drink again it is best practice to present only a very small portion of carefully selected food or drink at first. It is not a good idea, if you think someone is feeling sick, to ask '*do you feel sick?*', or '*are you going to vomit?*' This tends to make patients feel worse and to remain disinterested in trying some food and drink. It is more appropriate to just ask '*how are you feeling?*', and to allow the patient to respond.

Vomiting is always an unpleasant experience, both to do and to witness. If it happens in your presence remember to ensure privacy and dignity for the patient, to offer comforting words, and to help to clean the patient up afterward and to provide a suitable mouthwash. A patient who is nauseous can be prescribed an anti-emetic drug, which can be taken orally or given by injection. The registered nurse will administer this.

Diarrhoea

Another malfunction of the digestive system is diarrhoea. This may be caused by intestinal hurry in that peristalsis expels waste before the large intestine has time to reabsorb the water from the waste material which will

be passed out from the body as faeces. The result is loosely formed or liquid faeces. Again, this can lead to dehydration. The healthcare assistant must note the type and amount of faecal matter passed and record this on a fluid balance chart if one is in place, and in the nursing care plan.

Indigestion and heartburn

Patients sometimes complain of indigestion and/or heartburn. Medication can be prescribed to alleviate these troublesome symptoms, which can occur for several reasons, including the side effects of certain drugs. From a practical nursing aspect these can be related to the patient's position when eating and drinking, or how the patient actually manages the mechanics of eating and drinking. Nurses who physically feed patients need to take these factors into account.

Practical nursing aspects of nutrition

Most patients in hospital and at home eat perfectly normally for themselves. Patients who have intravenous infusions in place, or who are attached to monitoring equipment may be unsure as to how much or how far they can move their arms in order to eat and drink and therefore require a reassuring demonstration and explanation that they cannot damage anything. Make sure the tray of food and a drink is placed as close to them as possible. Patients who might need physical assistance with eating and drinking include those who have a dementia or are severely confused, anyone who is very frail, weak, or exhausted, or those who are severely depressed. Other patients who will require assistance are newly blinded people, or those having extensive bilateral eye surgery where they are blindfolded, spinally injured patients who have a paralysis of the arms, and patients who have extensive burns of the arms. Please note that we talk of assisting the patients with eating and drinking even though the healthcare assistant is physically feeding the patient. Assisting the patient to take food and drink, rather than the use of the term 'feeding' makes the patient feel more in control (it is after all the patient who is performing the acts of chewing and swallowing), and is part of the preservation of a patient's dignity.

The practical act of assisting patients who cannot eat and drink easily is a skilled competence. A good, safe technique is required which enables the patent to have a satisfactory experience.

- Prepare the immediate environment in which the patient is to receive food and drink. Is the table/locker top clean and tidy? Remove any old, used tissues for infection control purposes. Also remove, temporarily,

any urinals or commode chairs in the vicinity otherwise the patient is in effect eating in a toilet

- Ensure your patient does not need to go to the toilet beforehand. Patients who have a full bladder or who need to defecate will have their mind distracted by this so might bolt the food. Bolted food is less easily digested

- Ensure the patient is helped with hand washing facilities by taking a bowl of water, soap, and a towel to the patient. This should be done before a mealtime whether or not the patient has just been to the toilet, in line with a good infection control procedures

- Fresh smelling hands are pleasant to the patient so the healthcare assistant must also wash his/her own hands before feeding a patient

- Patients might not be able to anticipate what is going to be placed in the mouth, especially if they cannot see what is on the plate, so if the patient has not met you before, introduce yourself, say what you would like to do in helping the patient to enjoy a meal, and describe the food the patient is about to have. This is also a safety check that any foods the patient is allergic to, or dislikes, or cannot have on cultural grounds, is not about to be offered

- Place a mixture of the food on a spoon, or a fork (providing the patient does not have uncontrollable shaking) and inform the patient that you are just about to offer this so that the mouth is opened. We do not eat all our peas at once, followed by the meat, and then the potato, so a good tip is to put a mix of the food on a spoon or a fork, as you would like to have this offered to yourself

- Warn the patient if the food is hot. Give smaller mouthfuls of very hot or very cold food items

- Talk pleasantly to the patient because all nursing interactions should be appropriately social ones, and are not meant to be purely technical interventions. Do not say anything that requires a response when the patient is chewing because this makes the patient feel awkward and embarrassed. Be aware of the need to not overload the patient or distract him/her from a pleasurable experience with incessant chatter. Any conversation had is to be with the patient, and not with a colleague who might be sitting nearby assisting another patient to eat

- Tactfully observe for when the patient is ready to receive the next spoon/ forkful of food. Offer food at the pace the patient can manage, and not at your preferred pace. Some patients are slower to eat than others. If the ward is short of staff and there are many patients to feed then the registered nurse in charge of the ward that day should liaise in advance of the mealtime with the modern matron so that additional staff appear to help out

- Every few mouthfuls give elderly, frail patients a bit of a pause so that they do not become too exhausted
- Offer sips of a drink at sensible intervals between solid food being offered
- When offering drinks, if the patient is not using a straw, do not pour too much liquid into the patient's mouth, or pour too quickly as this causes a drowning sensation
- Ask the patient to say or indicate when he/she has had enough to eat and drink
- Never try to force-feed a patient. This is an assault. Seek advice and assistance from the registered nurse if a patient refuses to eat and/or drink.

Some patients receive their nutritional intake via routes other than the normal oral route, and therefore have liquid nutrition feed medically prescribed and dispensed by a pharmacy. Some have a surgical artificially created route, such as percutaneous endoscopic gastrostomy (PEG feeding), whilst other patients might have a naso-gastric nutrition regime. Healthcare assistants who are going to be involved in the care of these patients must receive training in the administration of these types of nutritional intake from a registered nurse, and competent performance must be signed-off before the healthcare assistant undertakes these duties on a solo basis.

Oral hygiene (mouth care)

Part of the mouth's structure also connects to the respiratory system, so problems arising in the mouth can, if allowed to go unnoticed or if not treated adequately, cause problems elsewhere in the body. In order to understand how these problems can occur and why mouth care (also known as oral toilet), is so important, there is a need to understand the structure of the mouth and the functions of its main components.

The mouth consists of two parts. The outer part is small, and is known as the vestibule. It is the space between the gums/teeth, and the lips/cheeks. The inner part is larger and is known as the oral cavity. This is the space behind the teeth and gums. The tongue is on the base of the oral cavity, and the hard palate ('roof of the mouth') forms the top. Towards the back of the oral cavity is the soft palate. The tonsils (if not surgically removed) will be found here at either side of the mouth, as will the uvula, a dangling but firmly fixed central structure, and from the soft palate are the respective openings into the trachea (the first part of the patient's airway), and the oesophagus (the gullet, the first part of the gastro-intestinal system). The salivary glands, of which there are three pairs, the parotid, situated just in front of each ear, the submandibular, situated just beneath the jaw line, and the sublingual, situated beneath the tongue, consist of sac-like alveoli, forming small lobules that lead into ducts which carry the salivary secretion into the mouth. Saliva is a watery, alkaline fluid containing ptyalin (salivary amylase) which acts on sugar and cooked starches. As well as having a chemical function, saliva also has a physical one. Saliva moistens the mouth, cleanses the tongue, makes speech easier (as those of you who have tried to speak with a dry mouth will know); and it lubricates food in the mouth, making swallowing easier. If a patient has a very dry mouth (xerostomia) due to an underlying physiological abnormality, or a disease process, the salivary glands may have ceased to function. Unfortunately, very ill and debilitated patients who receive inadequate mouth care also often develop this.

Food passes from the mouth to the oral pharynx, and from there to the laryngo-pharynx, which leads into the oesophagus. Attached to the lateral walls of the oral pharynx are the tonsils — collections of lymphoid tissue which help to guard against infection entering the gastrointestinal tract and the respiratory tract but in the course of doing so often become chronically infected themselves and may therefore surgically removed.

The structures and functions of the mouth are an important aid to ingesting fluids and therefore avoiding dehydration, and for digesting foodstuffs, which provide essential nutrients throughout the body.

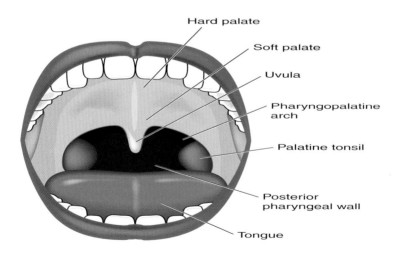

Figure 1. The structures of the mouth

Mastication, the act of chewing, is the biting and grinding of food between the upper and lower teeth. Movements of the tongue and cheeks assist until the food particle forms a small bolus which is pushed against the hard palate and then swallowed. Patients who have no teeth, or who have ill-fitting dentures, severe facial injuries, or those who have had a cerebral vascular incident (CVI, also known as a cerebral vascular accident, CVA, and commonly referred to as a stroke) will have difficulty with the normal mechanisms of eating and drinking and will require not only assistance with ingesting sufficient nutrients but also with oral hygiene. Patients who are likely to need assistance with mouth care are:

- Unconscious patients
- Those with facial injuries
- Stroke patients, especially where there are difficulties with speech and swallowing
- Those who are nil-by-mouth for significant periods of time
- Patients who are nil by mouth but being artificially fed e.g. by gastrostomies, or by intravenous infusion
- Immuno-suppressed patients, e.g. patients who have cancer or HIV. Patients receiving chemotherapy have particular oral hygiene needs to reduce the risk of mouth infections. Chemotherapy affects the ability to salivate so there is an increased risk of a build up of plaque.
- Patients with a low platelet count as they bleed easily even when brushing and flossing their teeth.

If a patient has a mouth problem that either goes unnoticed or is not adequately treated this is likely to mean that the patient will experience oral discomfort, may develop an inflammation of the mouth (stomatitis), or an infection of the mouth such as oral thrush (*Candida albicans*). Bad breath (halitosis) might also develop. Any one of these, let alone a combination of them, will mean the patient will be reluctant to eat and drink, and this very often leads to a cyclical problem where the original problem becomes worse and the patient's overall condition starts to decline as dehydration and malnutrition leads to a systemic weakness, which can be accompanied by a degree of reactive depression. Patients do not appreciate having a dirty mouth and cracked lips on top of their other health problems, and certainly do not like friends relatives to see them like this, especially if halitosis is present.

Thrush is a yeast fungus. It lives in the mouth and vagina of healthy persons but can cause illness in people with a weakened immune system when it affects the mouth, and if untreated can spread to the throat and the oesophagus. Thrush is usually treated with nystatin suspension on a 'swish and swallow' regime followed as prescribed by the doctor. The bottle and one dropper must be restricted to use by one named patient only to avoid the spread of infection. Make sure the dropper is rinsed thoroughly each time after use to avoid contaminating the contents of the suspension bottle.

Herpes simplex (mouth or cold sore) is a member of the herpes family of viruses. It is usually treated by the topical application (applied directly to the area) of acyclovir. Wear gloves if you are applying this and, again, confine use of the tube to the named patient.

Mouth care

Talk to the patient about why you would like to help them with mouth care, or perform mouth care for them. Unconscious patients can often hear what you say although they cannot respond so they should always be talked to and included in conversations. With conscious patients obtain their consent, trust and confidence. If you have any doubt about proceeding, check with a registered nurse first. The following procedure is for a fully co-operative patient. If the patient is agitated or is unable to co-operate consult the registered nurse about how to proceed. Some patients might benefit from having a close relative or loved one help perform mouth care. Talk to the relative or person concerned beforehand about this.

Gather the necessary equipment. This may vary according to where you work but will include the following type of materials: a clean plastic or cardboard tray the base of which is covered with a clean white paper towel or clean cloth, a small clean dish for water or a mouthwash, a denture pot (if required), a soft toothbrush (toothbrushes must be clean and in good condition and used for the same patient only), gauze swabs, toothpaste, lip balm or soft petroleum jelly, a small torch, tissues for wiping the mouth, gloves for your use, soft disposable forceps for gripping the gauze swabs, and a disposable paper bag for the used tissues.

A mouthwash is a product used for oral hygiene. Antiseptic and anti-plaque mouthwashes aim to remove plaque and the bacteria that proliferate on it, gingivitis (inflammation of the gums sometimes caused by infection), and halitosis. Anti-cavity mouthwashes use fluoride to help protect against tooth decay. However, this does not mean that brushing and flossing of the teeth should be neglected.

Mouthwashes are often acidic on the pH scale and because of this they should not be used for patients who are immuno-suppressed as the acidic content can wear away the oral mucosa. Use plain water for immuno-suppressed patients, or the brand of mouthwash prescribed by the doctor, checking with the registered nurse before use.

Other patients who would benefit from using plain water rather than a mouthwash with a high acidic content are those who have problems with heartburn, acid reflux, or indigestion. Oral hygiene (mouth care) procedure:

- Put on your gloves
- Ask the patient if he/she is experiencing any mouth discomfort. Ask the patient to open his/her mouth. If the patient is unconscious, gently open the mouth
- Inspect the mouth for any signs of inflammation or thrush. If the patient wears dentures check that these are not ill-fitting or loose and causing friction ulcers. If the dentures are a good fit but loose then consider using a firmer fixative as otherwise food substances can become trapped in between the denture and the gum causing discomfort and friction ulceration
- If the patient is not immuno-suppressed offer the toothpaste and toothbrush followed by either a glycothymoline mouthwash (the pink or green dissolvable tablets that dentists usually use) or plain water. If the patient's lips are dry then a proprietary lip balm or soft petroleum jelly can be applied. Do not use glycerine-based products as glycerine is hygroscopic meaning it draws water away from the lips, so whilst it leaves the lips looking moist this is a false impression because actually underneath the lips are getting drier.
- If the patient is unconscious or needs help dip the gauze swabs (do not use cotton wool balls as these tend to fluff and stick to the sides of the mouth, plus they are small and if your hand slips and loses its grip the cotton wool ball could find its way down the patient's airway!) into the mouthwash or clean water using either the soft, plastic forceps. Hold the dipped gauze swab between your thumb and first finger. Gently wipe the inside of the mouth one-way only. Using a fresh gauze swab each time, do this until the mouth looks clean. Do not reach too far into the back of the mouth, as this will cause the patient to gag
- Where the patient has teeth, apply toothpaste to the toothbrush and with gentle up and down movements clean the teeth. Wipe any excess toothpaste foam away with tissues and discard
- Apply lip balm or soft petroleum jelly
- If the patient is able to drink, with or without assistance, then offer a drink of the patient's choice
- The mouth care tray should be made up fresh for each use and on average this will be 2–4 hourly depending on the state of the patient's mouth
- Document the date and times mouth care is performed and record any concerns that you have about the condition of the patient's mouth, bringing this to the attention of the registered nurse
- It is important not to show any signs of revulsion even if the state of the patient's mouth and the halitosis is bad. Patients, even those who appear to neglect themselves, are often more aware and upset about their physical presentation than we think. We help patients with personal aspects of their hygiene not only to help prevent the incidence of infection, but in order to help preserve the patient's dignity, self-esteem, and a sense of their own unique identity.

Conclusion

As a general principle, it is also important and necessary to remind ourselves of the need to maintain high standards in respect of our own personal hygiene as there is nothing worse than being attended by someone with a strong body odour, which can include an overly strong deodorant, or perfume, or whose breath is not very fresh. It does tend to put you off wanting to eat and drink and by not paying attention to this area we do a disservice to our patients.

DH (2007a) <u>Hospital Food</u>. <u>http://www.dh.gov.uk/en/Managingyourorganisation/ Leadershipandmanagement/Healthcareenvironment/index.htm</u>. 4 October 2007.

DH (2007b) <u>Hospital Food</u>. <u>http://www.dh.gov.uk/en/Managingyourorganisation/ Leadershipandmanagement/Healthcareenvironment/</u> DH_4116450. 4 October 2007

CHAPTER 9

Elimination needs and catheter care

Sue Foxley

Most healthcare assistants working in primary care will see patients with continence problems every day but might not recognise that they have a difficulty with continence. This is because it is not usually the presenting problem and is likely to be in addition to existing health problems, possibly those of a chronic nature. The British Medical Association (2006) estimate that there are 17.5 million adults currently living with a long-term medical condition in the UK, many of those possibly are living in residential care home settings.

The demand for continence services has increased in recent years as a result of increased awareness and the inclusion of recommendations for improved continence care portrayed in the National Service Framework for Older People (DH, 2001). Continence will always remain a high priority amongst sufferers and their carers. With this in mind extra demands on nurses' time will be apparent. Nurses need to be encouraged to prioritise their workload as a continence assessment may be a low priority amongst other more pressing needs (Bayliss and Salter, 2004).

The main objective of continence care is to improve assessment, treatment and management of incontinence in health care, and to encourage collaboration and best practice amongst healthcare practitioners involved in continence care across primary and secondary care.

Political agenda

Thirteen years have passed since the Department of Health (1996) proposed the future of primary care services. An ambitious service would provide high quality, integrated health services, which were to be organised and run around the service users' needs. Despite the existence of a comprehensive NHS for over 60 years, many services remained disintegrated (Hands, 2001). Rising swiftly up the political agenda, firm foundations to improve practice were laid by the publication of *Good Practice in Continence Services* (DH,

2000) setting out a model of good practice to help achieve more responsive, equitable and effective continence care services across the country. Its main aim was to highlight the extent of the problem and set out clear, achievable targets for each service. Emphasis was placed upon the need to identify all people with incontinence in primary care and offer them an assessment by a suitably trained healthcare professional.

Prevalence of incontinence

Incontinence is not a newly discovered problem. It is not life threatening, but it certainly can be life changing (Haslam, 2005).

Gray (2005) suggests that there are common myths associated with incontinence that act as barriers for those wishing to seek help. Often a sufferer fails to consult with their GP, wrongly assuming that incontinence is a normal part of the ageing process (Continence Foundation, 1995) or as a consequence of childbirth (Newman, 2002). Jolley et al (1998) conducted a study to determine the reasons for under-reporting by patients, and these included embarrassment, belief that incontinence is a normal part of the aging process, availability of products for incontinence, poor knowledge regarding management options, low expectations regarding treatment, and fear of surgery.

A patient's quality of life is dependent on the availability of correct care facilities and individual patient-focused support. However, results from the first national audit of continence care in the UK (Royal College of Physicians, 2005) shows a widespread failure to diagnose and control continence problems effectively.

McGrother et al (2001) identified from the results of a systematic review of UK studies that there is strong evidence to confirm that incontinence is very common, more common than other chronic conditions such as asthma, diabetes and depression, and has a negative effect on quality of life (Milson et al, 2001). This is often distressing for the individual and represents a major public health problem that may increase over time.

The cost of incontinence

The economic burden of incontinence within the NHS is substantial, accounting for around 2% of the NHS budget (Wagg et al, 2003) and this will escalate as more people live longer (Parsons and Cardozo, 2004). The Continence Foundation (2000) estimated that in 1998 in England alone the cost of incontinence to the NHS was a minimum of £353 million. This figure rose to £420 million in 2000. Examining the economic issues surrounding incontinence, studies have revealed that substantial demands are currently placed upon NHS resources to manage the symptoms, despite highly effective and minimally invasive interventions being available (Lucas et al, 1999). Thomas (2001) advocates that savings can be made, however it is essential to derive the maximum return on the investment in better health.

An overview of urinary elimination

The International Continence Society (Ford-Martin and Frey, 2005) define urinary incontinence as the unintentional loss of urine which is sufficient enough in frequency and amount to cause the sufferer physical and emotional distress. Not medically classified as a disease, it is a symptom of lower urinary tract dysfunction which gives rise to problems which can be distressing and unpleasant for any sufferer (Kelly and Byrne, 2006).

Early reports of urinary incontinence date back to ancient Egyptian times. Ancient Greek medicine outlined several cures for incontinence, which originated from the work of Hippocrates in 460–377 BC. Gomez (2003) describes early remedies such as an infusion of white chrysanthemums in lukewarm water, or consuming a powder made from burnt cock's testicles. Alternatively, the sufferer could attach a frog to his belt. Getliffe and Dolman (2003) highlight the fact that it was during the nineteenth century the effect of certain food and drinks upon the bladder's function was identified.

Normal bladder function

The bladder is a hollow, balloon-shaped organ that is located in the pelvis (Parsons and Cardozo, 2004). It has two major functions: storage and emptying urine. Bladder control problems consist of conditions that affect either function (Norton, 2001).

The kidneys make urine all the time which constantly passes down the ureter's into the bladder (*Figure 1*). The bladder normally stores urine produced by the kidneys; it acts as a reservoir until the person finds a suitable convenient place and time to empty it (i.e. going to the toilet to pass urine).

Normal bladder function is heavily dependant upon several factors; these include fluid intake and lifestyle. The urinary bladder is primarily made up of muscle called the 'detrusor'. When this muscle contracts and the muscles in the urethra and pelvic floor relax the bladder empties. Complex nerve messages are sent between the brain, the bladder, and the pelvic floor muscles, telling the person when the bladder is ready to empty. If it is not convenient to pass urine the person should be able to hold on and stop the bladder from contracting until a convenient place is found. The ability to do this is usually learnt in childhood.

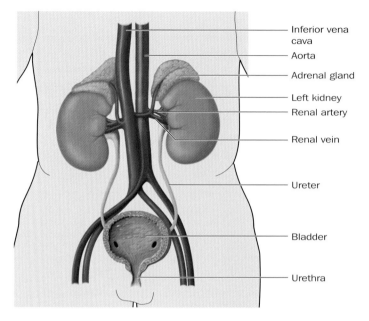

Figure 1 shows the anatomy of the bladder.

A guide to the classification of urinary incontinence, which can have an effect upon the patient's health and well being, is outlined in *Table 1*. Following extensive continence assessment, which is discussed at length later in this chapter, various treatment options can be discussed with the patient if deemed appropriate in their ongoing care. The healthcare assistant needs to be aware that a patient's bothersome urinary symptoms can be suppressed by various different treatments, although the underlying problem may not always be curable. *Table 2* outlines some of the treatments available. The healthcare assistant can ensure that the patient is aware of the recommendations shown in *Table 3* which could improve their bothersome bladder symptoms.

Effects on quality of life

Bothersome symptoms from bladder problems can certainly impede upon a person's quality of life. Effects and reactions to the symptoms can vary between individuals (Norton, 2003). The most bothersome problems a person with this condition can experience include:

- Increased visits to the general practitioner and time off work
- Fear of returning to work following a period of sickness for a continence related problem

Table 1.	Classification of urinary incontinence	
Type of incontinence	**Definition**	**Associated risk factors**
Stress	Involuntary leakage of urine on effort or exertion (e.g. coughing, sneezing)	Pregnancy, childbirth, obesity, pelvic surgery, chronic cough, race, genetic predisposition, collagen deficiency
Urge	Involuntary leakage of urine associated with or immediately preceded by urgency	Age, race, incontinence surgery, neurological conditions, childhood bed wetting
Mixed	Involuntary leakage associated with urgency and also with effort, exertion, coughing and sneezing	Age, race, incontinence surgery, neurological conditions, childhood bed wetting
Functional	Urinary incontinence where no organic cause can be found. May be due to cognitive or physical factors	Dementia, learning difficulties, immobility / disability, stool impaction, those in long-term institutions, medication
Overflow	Involuntary leakage associated with poor bladder emptying	Constipation, pelvic surgery, pregnancy, childbirth, bladder injury, pelvic organ prolapsed, neurological impairment, medication
Nocturnal enuresis	Involuntary leakage occurring during sleep	Developmental delay/ impairment, medication, sleep apnoea

Source: Rantell and Vosloo (2008)

Table 2.	Treatments for incontinence
• General lifestyle modifications	
• Bladder re-education and biofeedback	
• Medication	
• Pelvic floor muscle exercises	
• Complementary therapy	

- Increased risk of falls
- Increased risk of urinary tract infection
- Distress, embarrassment and lack of self-confidence
- Social isolation
- Expense of buying containment products
- Effect on personal relationships
- Dietary restrictions
- Sleep deprivation due to frequent visits to the toilet during the night.

Table 3. General lifestyle recommendations
a. Aim to drink 1–2 l of varied fluid a day
b. Occasionally people find that tea and coffee has a rapid diuretic effect (Norton, 2001)
c. Encourage the use of decaffeinated drinks
d. If the patient is taking diuretic medication ensure that they are aware how this medication works
e. Have their medication reviewed to ensure all is appropriate for their medical condition
f. Smoking is associated with urgency to void in older people (Dallosso et al 2003)
g. Educate the person regarding the most appropriate containment product use
h. Make getting to the toilet as easy for the person as possible - consider special adaptations
i. Only go to the toilet when the person needs to — avoid the 'just in case' scenario

Management

Management of such problems need to be addressed on an individual basis. It is clearly evident that healthcare assistants play a vital role in motivating and monitoring the patient.

Bladder re-education

Bladder training aims to restore the individual's confidence in the bladder's ability to hold urine and to re-establish a more normal pattern of voiding Norton (2001). Instead of rushing off to the toilet as soon as the person gets

the urge to pass urine (void), it is important to try and hold on. Learning to hold on can be a lengthy process, and the key to success is accurate record-keeping and professional support by a competent healthcare professional, who may well be a healthcare assistant.

It is imperative to establish how often the person currently voids, the healthcare assistant can be key to ensuring that collected documentation is accurate. Once a voiding pattern is established the person can increase the times between their trips to the toilet. Bladder re-education may take several forms:

- Timed voiding — whereby the person is encouraged to void at set times Habit training — this approach is an assigned toileting schedule for example two-hourly
- Prompted voiding — the person is prompted to void at regular or set intervals
- Promoting continence — involves a gradual increase in between voids
- Biofeedback — specialist treatment package only available from competent healthcare professionals. This method aims to teach patient's responses to improve bladder control (Bardsley, 2007).

Bladder re-education needs motivation, proper instruction and support from a competent healthcare professional, and this includes the healthcare assistant.

Medication

Medicines that calm a person's bladder down will allow them more time to get to the toilet. These are not designed as a course of tablets and therefore the person will need to obtain repeat prescriptions to maintain any benefit.

Medication of this type (antimuscarinics) are often started at a very low dose and gradually increased. This is to increase their efficacy and minimize their side effects. The most commonly used tablets are oxybutynin, tolterodine and solifenacin. These drugs are provided in a sustained-release formula, which means only taking it once a day. NICE (2006) provide guidance for healthcare professionals who prescribe medication for people with urinary incontinence.

In order for these particular drugs to be effective they are likely to cause some side effects, commonly a dry mouth, dry eyes, blurred vision and possibly constipation. Wagg et al (2007) highlight risks that are associated with prescribing medication for the older adult. However, there is a range of drugs that suit different patients but equally there is a certain amount of trial and error when trying to achieve success in treating patients' symptoms.

Pelvic floor muscle exercises

These exercises aim to strengthen the musculature of the pelvic floor. The pelvic floor is a group of muscles that plays a large part in maintaining continence. Not only do they act like a sling that supports the uterus, bladder and bowel, they also control the muscles of the urethral sphincter (bladder neck) and around the anal sphincter (back passage). By exercising the pelvic floor muscles the sphincters can be strengthened and therefore improve a person's continence.

A person needs to be very motivated to perform these exercises regularly so that they can achieve the best and quickest results. Ideally, an expert who can advise and support the person should teach pelvic floor exercises.

It is important to remember that exercising the pelvic floor muscles is for life. If a patient fails to comply with this management option it is likely that any weakness will return and problems with leakage may return.

Complementary therapy

Several different therapies have been found effective in the treatment of an overactive bladder. Two examples are listed below:

- Hypnotherapy (Freeman, 1989)
- Acupuncture (Vosloo, 2007).

Surgical intervention

There are many surgical procedures available to treat urinary incontinence. For stress incontinence these include mid urethral tapes, colposuspension, and urethral bulking agents. Overflow incontinence caused by urethral strictures can be relieved by urethral dilatation or urethrotomy. For urge incontinence injection of Botox into the detrusor muscle has been found to be effective. In extreme cases urinary diversion may be necessary. It is essential to be aware of all the risks and benefits before a patient undergoes surgery.

An overview of bowel elimination

Caring for patients who experience bowel dysfunction is a common feature of clinical nursing practice, and for some patients this is essential to their medical management. Bowel dysfunction can be a symptom which can be caused by an underlying anatomical or functional problem. The term constipation can mean different things to different people. It can be a feeling

of difficulty of passing stool, accompanied by excessive straining, or a complaint of infrequent bowel movements. Frequency of bowel movement varies widely in the population, and it is considered normal to pass stools between three times a day and three times a week. Faecal incontinence which affects up to one in 10 of the population at any given time involves the involuntary loss of wind, liquid or stool (Powell, 2008).

Defining constipation

Powell and Rigby (2000) indicate that people with constipation do not present with distinctive symptoms. Many patients will use the term constipation to describe difficult passage of a hard formed stool or a feeling of not completely emptying their bowel. There is a wide range of causes of constipation which will be outlined later. The healthcare assistant needs to ensure that they are fully aware of each of the possible causes. *Table 4* outlines the international classification of constipation used by healthcare professionals.

Normal bowel function

The bowel is part of the digestive system which starts in the mouth and finishes in the anus. The role of the digestive system is to digest the food we consume daily, absorb the good nutrients and expel the waste products no

---

Table 4.   **A diagnosis of constipation needs to include two or more of the following:**

- Straining during at least 25% of defecations

- Lumpy or hard stools in at least 25% of defecations

- Sensation of incomplete evacuation for at least 25% of defecations

- Sensation of ano-rectal obstruction/blockage for at least 25% of defecations

- Manual removal of stool in at least 25% of defecations

- Less than three defecations per week

- Loose stools are rarely present without laxative use

- Insufficient criteria to diagnose Irritable bowel syndrome.

Source: Longstreth et al (2006)

---

longer required by the body. The colon, or large bowel, absorbs fluid from this waste as it is passing through, moved along with rhythmic contractions of the bowel (peristalsis), to gradually form it into stools (also known as faeces and bowel motions). The stools are then stored in the rectum at the end of the large bowel until they is expelled. A complex system of sensitive nerve endings allow the patient to know whether it is wind, loose stool or normal stool in the rectum, and whether they can safely release it or contract the muscles around the anus to hold it in.

Normal defaecation

Norton (2001) describes the process of rectal emptying which is usually initiated voluntarily. Movement of faeces into the rectum causing rectal distension evokes the desire to defaecate, known as the 'call to stool'. Under the appropriate circumstances defaecation is completed when the person adopts a sitting or squatting position that allows abdominal pressure to rise by contraction of the diaphragm and abdominal muscles, followed by relaxation of the puborectalis muscle and external anal sphincter muscles stool is then expelled.

Stool production and what influences this

Healthcare assistants need to be aware that patients will experience the urge to open their bowels a few minutes after they have had a meal and this is due to massive contractions of the colon triggered by food reaching the stomach.

Normal stool output per day is around 200g. The upper colon defines the consistency and volume of delivery of contents to the rectum. Bowel frequency in a healthy person may vary between 1–3 times a day to 3 times a week, and is influenced by gender, diet and health (Norton and Chelvanayagam, 2004). Stool consistency can vary (see *Figure 2*).

Possible causes of bowel dysfunction

These can be divided into two main groups then further sub-divided. A full continence assessment undertaken by a competent healthcare professional will help to identify the patient's problem:

1. Functional problems
2. Anatomical problems

Functional problems

Medications: Some prescribed or over the counter medications can cause bowel dysfunction as a side-effect. These can include painkillers, iron tablets, anti-depressants, tablets used to treat bladder problems and some medications for lowering high blood pressure (Eberhardie, 2003).

A poor diet and not enough exercise: The intake of refined and rich food, lacking in vitamins and minerals, as well as hurried eating, insufficient chewing, eating large quantities of meat and the wrong combination of foods can all play a

Type 1	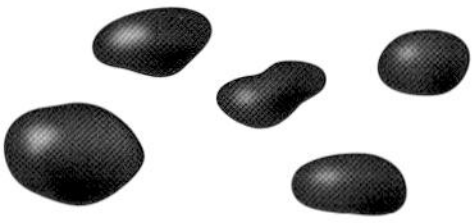	Separate hard lumps, like nuts (hard to pass)
Type 2	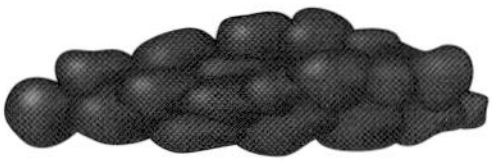	Sausage-shaped but lumpy
Type 3	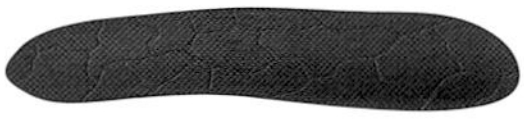	Like a sausage but with cracks on its surface
Type 4	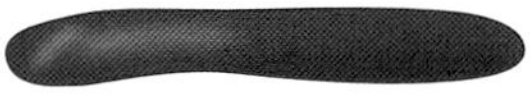	Like a sausage or snake, smooth and soft
Type 5	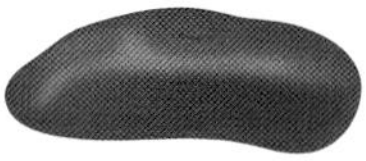	Soft blobs with clear cut edges (passed easily)
Type 6	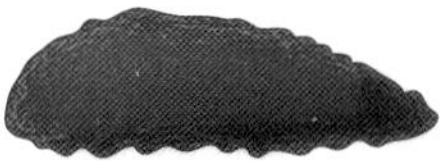	Fluffy pieces with ragged edges, a mushy stool
Type 7	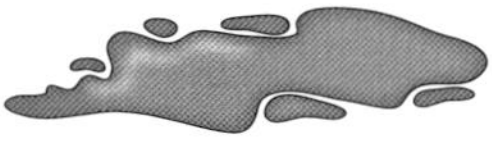	Watery, no solid pieces. Entirely liquid

Figure 2. The Bristol stool scale showing different stool consistencies.

role in influencing stool formation which can lead to bowel dysfunction. A lack of regular exercise and weak abdominal muscles are associated risk factors (Joanna Briggs Institute, 1999; Haggar, 1998).

Lifestyle and bowel habits: Failure to respond to the urge to open your bowels and delay in passing stool slows the gut and results in bowel dysfunction. This may happen when away on holiday, or when a person does not feel comfortable using a public toilet. More often than not people are too busy to respond to the call to stool.

Environmental factors: The healthcare assistant will be able to play a very important role in monitoring if environmental factors are causing any problems for the patient presenting with bowel dysfunction. For example: poor toileting facilities, incorrect positioning on the toilet/commode, lack of privacy, lack of nursing/social care, fear of the need of the patient to perform on demand, restricted clothing, distance to the toilet, use of bedpans, and lack of signage. More often than not these environmental factors are easily resolved.

Pregnancy and after childbirth: Anderson (1986) suggests that hormonal changes during pregnancy and whilst breastfeeding can slow the gut and cause constipation. New mothers are often very busy and do not allow themselves the time to respond to the urge to open their bowels. Slowing their gut by putting off the urge results in constipation (Marshall et al, 1996). Healthcare assistants need to be aware of this fact when working in this care setting.

Menstrual cycle: One in six women suffer with constipation in the second half of their menstrual cycle and this is linked with dietary changes caused by premenstrual tension (Rees and Rhodes, 1976).

Eating disorders: Healthcare assistants need to ensure that their patients eat regularly otherwise they will not have a normal bowel action. Screening of a patient's nutritional state is an essential requirement of all health care personnel (DH, 2001). Anorexia nervosa and bulimia are two extreme examples of eating disorders you need to be aware of. Leddy (2007) highlights the abuse of laxatives by those people with an eating disorder.

Following an operation: Normal bowel contractions can be markedly reduced following abdominal surgery, and some patients may put off the urge to have their bowels moved as it is too painful to push. A general anaesthetic and painkillers given after any operation can slow down the gut's motility, leading to bowel dysfunction.

The normal colon has five main functions	
STORAGE	The colon stores unabsorbed food residue. Within 72 hours, 70% of this has been excreted. The remaining 30% can stay in the colon for up to a week
ABSORPTION	Sodium, water, chloride, some vitamins, drugs including steroids and aspirin are absorbed from the colon
SECRETION	Mucus is secreted and used to lubricate the faeces
SYNTHESIS	Vitamins – a small amount of vitamin K is produced
ELIMINATION	Through peristaltic movement of the faecal matter into the rectum. Its presence is detected by sensory nerve endings a sensation of fullness is experienced, followed by a desire to defecate.
	Norton (2001)

A fear of pain: Haemorrhoids and anal fissures can cause pain and bleeding on passing stool and in turn cause constipation to develop.

Psychological disturbances: Bowel dysfunction is common in those people under much stress, or in those who suffer from depression and anxiety (Longsttreth et al, 2006).

Psychiatric problems: Healthcare assistants need to appreciate that those patients with depression, confusion and dementia may be susceptible to constipation. Equally, constipation may be an underlying factor of a patient that presents with confusion. It is important to monitor bowel actions in 'at risk' patient groups. The healthcare assistant can take the lead on this, ideally reporting any problem to trained healthcare personnel.

Anatomical problems

Rectocele

A bulging of the rectum into the vagina, called a rectocele or posterior vaginal wall prolapse can create a pouch where stool can become trapped. Patients often experience difficulty in passing stool, straining and a feeling of incomplete emptying of the rectum. In these cases the patient will perform vaginal or anal digitation (inserting a finger into the vagina/anus/rectum to assist defaecation) (Emmanuel, 2004).

Diseases and injuries

The healthcare assistant needs to be aware of the abundant diseases and injuries that can predispose to constipation, for example: Hirschsprungs disease, mega colon, spinal injury, neurological disease for example multiple sclerosis, large bowel carcinoma, haemorrhoids, anal stricture, anal fissure, endocrine disorders for example diabetes mellitus and diverticular disease.

Symptoms and complications of constipation

All healthcare personnel need to be aware that bowel dysfunction can cause distressing symptoms for the patient such as abdominal bloating, generalised pain, nausea and vomiting, general malaise, loss of appetite, sudden or worsening urinary incontinence and rectal discomfort. Constant straining to move stool can lead to haemorrhoids which can be painful and even bleed on passing stool. If bodily waste is not eliminated from the body effectively, toxic build-up can lead to further problems like headaches and mood swings. Symptoms of low back pain, heartburn, bad breath and a coated tongue can also be experienced by the patient.

Treatment options

The ideal management of bowel dysfunction involves identification and if possible elimination of the primary cause. Education of the patient in the physiology of defaecation, initiation of a good diet and if appropriate laxatives to be used until bowel function is restored (Wiesel et al, 2001). General advice regarding lifestyle, bowel habits and the importance of regular exercise is essential and can be given by the healthcare assistant.

An overview of urinary catheter care

A urinary catheter is a hollow tube which is inserted into the bladder, either for intermittent or permanent use. The catheter tube is designed to enable drainage of urine from the bladder, or for instillation of medication directly into the bladder's cavity. It is associated with significant morbidity and mortality and should be avoided if at all possible (Tew et al, 2005). Where it is necessary healthcare assistants should meet the required performance criteria and possess the necessary complex skills and knowledge to ensure safe and effective management of the care bundle for urinary catheters and appliances.

Indications for urinary catheterisation

Urinary catheterisation can be one of the important aspects of the holistic care bundle patients receive. Indications for the patient having to undergo this procedure are outlined in *Table 5*. It is worth noting that urinary catheterisation should never be used for nursing convenience, patients should not be catheterised routinely there must always be a valid reason for this procedure to be undertaken.

Identifying best practice in urinary catheter care

The literature clearly defines that a high percentage of patients admitted to hospital are catheterised unnecessarily (Pomfret, 2006; Stewart, 2006). Pratt et al (2007) advocate that urinary catheterisation should not be undertaken unless it is medically required, and even then the catheter should remain in place for as short as time as possible.

Long standing debate continues within the nursing profession around best practice in the management of urinary catheters (Norton, 2001; Getliffe and Dolman, 2003; Dougherty and Lister, 2004, RCN, 2008).

Interestingly Rawlinson and Clark (2004) suggest that best practice in the management of indwelling catheters is achieved by the healthcare assistant gaining basic knowledge of the makes of catheter and disposable urinary drainage bags available. Whilst best practice is advocated, it is not embedded into clinical practice therefore accessing and appraising evidence is rapidly becoming a core clinical competency and clinical decisions can no longer be based on opinion alone.

Catheter related procedures undertaken by a competent healthcare assistant

Healthcare assistants may undertake a range of catheter care procedures following patient assessment by a qualified competent nurse. If he or she has been deemed competent in the particular catheter care task and that the employing organisation permits them to perform that particular task, the qualified nurse can agree to delegate that task to that particular healthcare assistant having gained the patient consent. The healthcare assistant should work as the patient's advocate in all aspects throughout urinary catheter care. *Table 6* outlines when it is acceptable for the following procedures / tasks to be undertaken by a competent healthcare assistant on a named patient basis.

Evaluation of competency

Acceptable performance criteria for the healthcare assistant's clinical practice should be met through observation and supervision by competent qualified nursing staff. This needs to be documented and counter signed by the supervisory nurse and kept within the healthcare assistant's personal portfolio. Urinary catheter care more often than not can be most problematic for patient and carer, these needs to be appreciated by all healthcare assistants.

Table 5.	Indications for catheterisation
Drainage	Critical care • Acutely paralysed bladder • Accurate measurement of output in severe illness • Monitoring of fluid balance
	Chronic retention • Incomplete bladder emptying • Decompression of chronic urinary retention • To bypass obstruction — prostate enlargement/urethral strictures • Uterine fibroids/abdominal mass
	Acute care • Pre and post operatively • Acute urinary retention • Over distension injury to the bladder • Neurological problems — disc protrusion/tumour
Management	Short and long term • Clean intermittent self catheterisation by a patient who has been taught to undertake this procedure
	• Supra pubic catheterisation as an alternative to urethral catheterisation
Investigation	• To perform urodynamic investigation • To measure residual urine — if bladder scan unavailable
Instillation	• Instillation of drugs • Catheter maintenance solutions
Intractable Incontinence	• End of life care • Pressure ulcers
Catheterise only as a last resort, when all other methods of bladder management have been tried and failed.	

Continence assessment

The success of treating bladder and bowel problems relies on a complete and effective continence assessment undertaken by a competent professional.

Why should we perform continence assessment?

An assessment is an essential part of the initial management of the patient that presents with a containment problem. Assessment establishes a presumed

Table 6. **Catheter care a trained healthcare assistant may carry out**
• Empty a urinary catheter bag or valve
• Form / connect and disconnect a link system
• Wash a patient with an indwelling catheter, including meatal care (DH, 2007)
• Move a patient with an indwelling catheter in line with local policies on manual handling
• Be aware of and use a variety of catheter care support equipment
• Change a catheter bag or valve aseptically
• Remove an indwelling Foley urethral catheter
• Insert an indwelling catheter where this is deemed to be low risk
• Classify if a situation is serious
• Administer a catheter maintenance solution
• Undertake urinalysis, obtain a specimen of urine and send for culture
• Identify and interpret the signs and symptoms of a catheter associated urinary tract infection
• Maintain appropriate bag positions
• Educate the patient about catheter care
• Accurately document all patient care performed
• Reporting, liaising and communication — inform the qualified nurse of any problems / concerns about the patient
• Order appropriate catheter care equipment
• Be aware that some equipment needs to conform with CE (kite mark) safety and maintenance requirements
RCN (2008)

aetiology and identifies complex cases (Ballentyne, 2005). This enables all healthcare professionals to offer the appropriate patient management and treatment. When containment problems occur most people go to see their GP or their practice nurse in their local surgery, seeking advice on management options. Ongoing care is likely to be organised through their GP and the primary care team. Clearly this type of continence problem is very common therefore can be treated effectively in primary care (Wilkinson, 2005).

It has been shown that patient empowerment is the most dynamic, effective and efficient approach to care (Addison, 2000). This places choices and decisions into the hands of those with incontinence. Wilkinson (2006) suggests that the first step to a diagnosis of urinary incontinence is for a continence assessment to be undertaken, followed by initiating appropriate treatment and formulating a management plan with the patient.

Assessment can be defined as the collection of raw data which is both objective and subjective (Ballentyne, 2005); this is viewed as the most vital stage in the nursing process which underpins essential nursing care (Allport, 1995). Key components of a continence assessment which may be started

---

Table 7. Key components of a continence assessment

• Review of symptoms and their effect on quality of life

• Assessment of the patient's desire for treatment and possible alternative management

• Examination of the patient's abdomen for palpable mass or retention of urine

• Examination of the perineum to identify prolapse, excoriation and assess pelvic floor contraction

• Rectal examination to exclude faecal impaction

• Urinalysis to exclude urinary tract infection

• Assessment of manual dexterity

• Assessment of the patient's environment–access to the toilet / use of toileting aids.

• Use of a bladder diary: frequency/volume chart, bladder scan

• Containment product review

• Identification of conditions that may exacerbate the patient's incontinence — medication, coughs, drinking habits, smoking, and bowel habit

(DH, 2000)

---

by a competent healthcare assistant are outlined in *Table 8*. These key components are grouped into four distinctive headings which are classified as history taking, physical examination, urine testing and contributory factors.

Healthcare professionals with a demonstrated competency are ideally placed to carry out level one assessment, each providing their own contribution to effective continence management, thus demonstrating that healthcare assistants play a valuable role in continence assessment.

Conclusion

Incontinence is a common clinical problem. To suffer from any form of incontinence is a demeaning and distressing experience that merits evidence-based care and an understanding by all healthcare personnel. Accurate continence assessment initiated by the healthcare assistant will help determine the extent of the problem and reveal the impact of bothersome symptoms on the person's quality of life. If incontinence is approached in a systematic manner it possibly can be remedied in most, if not all, sufferers.

Addison R (2000) Fluid Intake: how coffee and caffeine affect continence. *Nursing Times* **96**(4): 7–8

Allport C, Campell J, Swain MAP (1995) A theoretical approach to nursing assessment. *Journal of Advanced Nursing* **10:** 111–5

Anderson AS (1986) Dietary factors in the aetiology and treatment of constipation during pregnancy. *British Journal of Obstetrics and Gynaecology* **93**(3): 245–9

Ballentyne M (2005) Assessment, Nursing Models and Best Practice. In: Addison R ed. *Nurse Led Continence Clinics*. Coloplast Ltd, Peterborough

Bardsley A (2007) Treating overactive bladder and urinary incontinence. *Continence UK* **1**(1): 22–8

Bayliss V, Salter L (2004) Pathways for evidence- based continence care. *Nursing Standard* **19**(9): 45–51

Bonner L (2005) Behavioural and lifestyle interventions and best practice. In: Addison R ed. *Nurse Led Continence Clinics*. Coloplast Ltd, Peterborough: 125–41

British Medical Association (2006) Health Policy Review. Published summer 2006. Available (Online) www.bma.org.uk. Accessed 6th May 2008

Brown JS, Vittinghoff E, Wyman JF et al (2000) Urinary incontinence: does it increase risk for falls and fracture? Study of Osteoporotic Fractures Research Group. *Journal American Geriatric Society* **48**: 721–5

Catherin M (2006) Saint Catherine of Alexandria Virgin, Martyr C. 310 AD (Online) Available at www.ewtn.com (accessed 15TH May 2008)

Colley W (2008) Five essential interventions in urinary incontinence care. *Continence Essentials* **1:** 40–3

Continence Foundation (CF) (1995) *Charter for Continence*. Continence Foundation, London

Continence Foundation (2000) *Making the Case for Investment in an Integrated Continence Service*. Continence Foundation, London

Cravens D, Zweig S (2000) Urinary catheter management. *American Academy of Family Physicians* **61**(2): 369–76

Dallosso HM, McGrother CW, Matthews RJ, Donaldson MK, Leicestershire MRC Incontinence Study Team (2003) The association of diet and other lifestyle factors with overactive bladder and stress incontinence; a longitudinal study in women. *British Journal Urology International* **92:** 67–7

Department of Health (1996) *The NHS, A Service with Ambitions*. DH, London

Department of Health (2000) *Good Practice in Continence Services*. DH, London

Department of Health (2001) *Essence of Care: Patient- focused Benchmarking for Healthcare Practitioners*. DH, London

Department of Health (2005) *National Standards, Local action, Health and Social Care Standards and Planning Framework*. DH, London

Department of Health (2007) *Saving Lives-High Impact Intervention No 6, Urinary catheter care bundle*. DH, London

Doughty DB (2000) *Urinary and Faecal Incontinence: Nursing Management*. Mosby, London

Dougherty L, Lister S (2004) *The Royal Marsden Manual of Clinical Nursing Procedures* 6th edn. Blackwell Publishing, London

Eberhardie C (2003) Constipation: identifying the problem. *Nursing Older People* **15**(9): 22–6

Emmanuel A (2004) Constipation. In: Norton C, Chelvanayagam S (2004) Bowel Continence Nursing. Beaconsfield Publishers Ltd, Buckinghamshire: 238–50

Euro Monitor (2001) *World Survey of Incontinent Products*. Euro Monitor, London

Evans D (2008) Managing continence issues in the workplace. *Continence Essentials* **1:** 16–21

Fleming A, Day J, Glanfield L (2000) Registered nurse management of urinary catheters in a rehabilitation and long-term care hospital. *International Journal of Nursing Practice* **6**(5): 237–45

Freeman RM (1989) Hypnosis and psychomedical treatment. Chapter 10. In: Freeman R, Malvern J eds. *The Unstable Bladder*. London

Ford–Martin P, Frey P (2005) Urinary Incontinence. Published 25th October 2005. Available online www.keepmedia.com. Accessed 6th May 2008

Getliffe K, Dolman M (1997 and 2003) Promoting Continence, A Clinical and Research Resource. Bailliere Tindall, London

Glynn A, Ward V, Wilson J, Charlett , Cookson B, Taylor L, Cole, N (1997) *Hospital – Acquired Infection: Surveillance, Policies and Practice*. Public Health Laboratory Service, London

Gray M (2005) Introduction Quality Care, A quarterly newsletter from the National Association for Continence. 23(4). Charleston SC: NAFC

Gomez J (2003) *Coping with Incontinence*. Sheldon Press, London

Haggar V (1998) Understanding Constipation. *Journal of Nursing Care*. **Summer:** 11–3

Hands D (2001) Integrated Care. In Lugon M, Secker-Walker J eds. *Clinical Governance: Making it Happen* eds. The Royal Society of Medicine Press Ltd, London

Haslam J (2005) Urinary Incontinence: Why women do not ask for help. *Nursing Times* **101**(47): 47–8

Joanna Briggs Institute (1999) Management of constipation in older adults. *Best Practice* **3**(1): 1–6

Jolleys JJ et al (1994) Urinary symptoms in the community; how bothersome are they? *British Journal of Urology* **74:** 551–5

Kelly AM, Byrne G (2006) Role of the continence nurse in health promotion. *British Journal of Nursing* **15**(4): 198–204

Leddy J (2007) Continence issues in laxative abuse and eating disorders. *Continence UK* **1**(3): 17–21

Longstreth G, Grant Thompson W, Chey W, Houghton L, Mearin F, Spiller R (2006) Functional bowel disorders. *Gastroenterology* **130:** 1480–91

Lucas M, Emery S, Beyon J (1999) *Incontinence*. Blackwell Science Ltd, Oxford

Marshall K, Totterdal D, McConnell V, Walsh DM, Whelan M (1996) Urinary incontinence and constipation during pregnancy and childbirth. *Physiotherapy* **82**(2): 98–103

McGrother CW, Shaw CI, Dallosso SM, Mensah FK (2001) Epidemiology (Europe). In: Cardoxo L, Staskin D eds. Textbook of Female Urology and Urogynaecology. Oxford: Isis Medical Media. 21–5

Milson I et al (2001) How Widespread are Symptoms of an Overactive Bladder and How are they Managed? A Population-based Prevalence Study. *British Journal of Urology International* **87:** 760–6

Murphy LJT (1972) *The History of Urology*. Charles C Thomas, Springfield

Newman D (2002) *Managing and Treating Urinary Incontinence*. Health Professions Press, Maryland

NICE (2006) *Urinary Incontinence: the management of urinary incontinence in women.*

NICE, London

Norton C (2001) *Nursing for Continence* 2nd edn. Beaconsfield Publishers, Beaconsfield

Norton C (2003) OAB evidence from the patient's perspective. *European Urology* **2**(Suppl 5): 16–22

Norton C, Chelvanayagam S (2004) *Bowel Continence Nursing*. Beaconsfield Publishers Ltd, Buckinghamshire

O'Brien J, Austin M, Sethi P, O'Boyle P (1991) Urinary incontinence: prevalence, need for treatment and effectiveness of intervention by nurse. *British Medical Journal* **303**: 1308–12

Parsons M, Cardozo L (2004) *Female Urinary Incontinence*. Royal Society of Medicine Press Ltd, London

Pomfret I (2006) Which urinary system is for you? *Charter Continence Care* **4**: 12–3

Powell M, Rigby D (2000) Management of bowel dysfunction: evacuation difficulties. *Nursing Standard* **14**(47): 47–51

Powell M (2008) The mechanics and assessment of faecal incontinence. *Continence UK* **2**(2): 40–3

Pratt RJ, Pellowe CM, Wilson JA et al (2007) epic 2: National evidence-based guidelines for preventing healthcare-associated infections in NIIS hospitals in England. *Journal of Hospital Infection* **65**(Suppl 1): S1–S64

Quick Reference Guide 14 (2000) Continence assessment. *Nursing Standard* **14**: 24

Rantell A, Vosloo R (2008) Urinary continence management in women. *Practice Nursing* **19**(5): 1–5

Rawlinson M, Clarke J (2004) Alternative approaches to managing a non-draining catheter. *British Journal of Community Nursing* **9**(4): 12–4

Rees WDW, Rhodes JWT (1976) Altered bowel habit and menstruation. *Lancet* **1**(7982): 475

Royal College of Nursing (2008) *Catheter Care*. RCN, London

Royal College of Physicians (2005) National Audit of Continence Care. Published 23rd November 2005 (Online) Available at www.rcplondon.ac.uk. 7TH May 2008

Shah J, Leach G (2001) *Urinary Incontinence*. Health Press Limited, Oxford

Stewart E (2006) Development of catheter care guidelines for Guy's and St Thomas'. *British Journal of Nursing* **15**(8): 420–5

Tew L, Pomfret I, King D (2005) Infection risks associated with urinary catheters. *Nursing Standard* **20**(7): 55–61

Thomas S (2001) Continence in Older People: a priority for primary care. *Nursing Standard* **15**(25): 45–50

Vosloo R (2007) Acupuncture for incontinence-what is the evidence? *Continence Review Plus*. Amber Educational Ltd, London: 8–9

Wagg A, Chapple C, Kirby M, Wells M (2003) The National Service Framework for Older People: Achieving the Standard in Continence Care. A Prescriber Supplement. Pfizer Ltd

Wagg A, Cardozo L, Chapple C, De Ridder D, Kelleher C, Kirby M, Milsom I, Vierhout M the Overactive Bladder Faculty (2007) Overactive bladder syndrome in older people. *British Journal Urology International* **99**(3): 502–9

Wagner TH, Hu TW, Bentkover J, LeBlanc K, Stewart W, Corey R, Zhou Z, Hunt T (2002) Health-related consequences of overactive bladder. *American Journal of Management Care* **8**(19): S598–607

Weisel PH, Norton C, Brazzelli M (2001) Management of faecal incontinence and constipation in adults with central neurolgical diseases. Cochrane Database of Systematic Reviews. Issue 1, 4, CD002115

Wilkinson K (2006) Urinary Incontinence. *Women's Health* **1**(1): 43–4

CHAPTER 10

Managing pain and providing comfort

Carol Haigh

The purpose of this chapter is to explore the issues of pain management and the role of the healthcare assistant in the recognition, assessment and treatment of pain. A working definition of pain will be presented, together with an overview of the tools available for the assessment and recording of pain and an outline of the strategies available to the healthcare worker to address or alleviate the patient's pain experience. The latter part of the chapter will be an examination of the concept of 'comfort' and will explore how the provision of comfort can impact upon the pain management of the patient.

What is pain?

Although most of us have experienced pain to a greater or lesser degree, actually coming up with a clear definition of what pain is and, more importantly, understanding what pain means to others, is extremely difficult. Part of this difficultly is because as well as the physical response the meaning that is given to pain varies from person to person. How an individual feels about their pain, how it impacts on their social roles and how they choose to behave when experiencing it is so personal that healthcare providers often find this the greater challenge when managing pain. Pain means different things to different people and it is very difficult to clearly classify it. We know that it is often associated with some form of tissue damage and most of the definitions of pain tend to concentrate upon that. For example:

> '...an unpleasant sensory or emotional experience associated with actual or potential tissue damage, or described in terms of such damage'.
> International Association for the Study of Pain (1986)

Other definitions prefer to take a simpler viewpoint:

'Pain is whatever the experiencing person says it is and exists whenever they say it does'.

McCaffery and Beebe (1994)

Unfortunately the first definition can be seen as too simplistic, since it ignores all of the other factors that may contribute to pain in an individual. The second one is very popular with nurses but does have a weakness since it rarely translates into appropriate managements of an individual's self reported pain. This is because very few nurses are willing to believe patients when they say they are in pain, preferring to put professional experience over patient reality (Carr and Mann, 2000). The important things to remember about any type of pain are:

- It is different things to different people
- It is something that cannot be ignored
- One of the key elements of good pain management is assessment.

It can be argued that managing pain is more important than defining it. However, because different types of pain require different types of management it is important that there is some understanding of the cause and the mechanisms of a patient's pain. The type of pain experienced by a patient not only affects the sort of treatment used but also the type of pain assessment carried out.

Types of pain

Broadly speaking there are three main types of pain. Each type has a different cause and way of assessing it, although often the same sort of treatment can be used.

Acute pain

Acute pain is usually recognised to be pain from injury (including surgery) or pain due to disease like toothache or heart attack. It is generally intense, localised to a specific area and is time limited in that as the injury heals or the disease abates the pain lessens. Acute pain can come from bone, joints, muscle, skin or connective tissue. It can also occur in visceral organs such as the gut or the pancreas. It can be sharp, stabbing, aching or throbbing in quality and is well localised.

How can acute pain be managed? This pain responds well to drug therapy. Drugs, known as analgesics, work well to mange this pain. There are different types of analgesia which have increasing pain relieving properties; non-opioid drugs like paracetamol, weak opioids such as codeine and strong opioids like morphine.

There are a number of problems associated with drug therapy, particularly with the opioid and opioid-type drugs such as nausea and vomiting and constipation. However, one of the biggest obstacles to the satisfactory management of acute pain is fear of addictions. Some patients and a considerable number of nurses are afraid of the opiate class of drugs, fearing that they will cause addiction. Whilst the opiate drugs do have the capacity to cause addiction if used recreationally, the risk of becoming dependent upon them, particularly when being used in acute pain management, is so small it is insignificant (Ferrall et al, 1992). Fear of addiction should *never* be used as a reason for not managing acute pain properly.

Chronic pain

Chronic pain is generally accepted to be pain that lasts for a long period of time, lasting beyond the time of healing of an injury and often there is no identifiable cause or explanation for it (International Association for the Study of Pain, 1986). It is associated with abnormal processing of sensory input by the peripheral or central nervous system, so unlike acute pain — which is initiated by trauma or chemical stimulus — chronic pain is allied to abnormal processing of information. Chronic pain can be described as centrally generated or peripherally generated pain. Centrally generated pain is associated with injury to either the peripheral or central nervous system. For example phantom limb pain may reflect injury to the peripheral nervous system. Peripherally generated pain relates to painful neuropathies. In patients who suffer from these, pain is felt along the distribution of many peripheral nerves. It is often bilateral and always diffuse. It can be caused by metabolic disturbances or toxic agents, for example diabetic neuropathy. Unlike acute pain which is initiated by chemical release, chronic pain is reliant upon 'abnormal' action of the nervous system.

How can chronic pain be managed? Unlike acute pain, chronic pain is not generally responsive to opioids in the long term so treatment usually includes different analgesics. Quite a number of the drugs that are used to manage acute pain are also used to manage the early stages or the occasional 'flare up' of chronic pain. Although alternate and complementary therapies can be used with acute pain to good effect, such therapies are often secondary approaches designed as adjuncts to drug therapy. However, in chronic pain management treatments such as relaxation, imagery, exercise, hypnosis, complementary therapies and disciplines such as physiotherapy, clinical

psychology and counselling used either on their own or in conjunction with analgesia and other drug therapies to control or reduce the patient's chronic pain form a more substantial part of the pain management plan. A further distinction between acute pain and chronic pain is that whereas acute pain is in the most part completely or significantly reduced by treatment, chronic pain may prove more intractable and difficult to cope with. Sometime the best that can be achieved is a slight reduction in the pain and when this is the case the treatment focus moves to coping strategies instead.

Pain associated with palliative care

Palliative care is defined as any form of medical care or treatment that concentrates on reducing the severity of disease symptoms, rather than striving to halt, delay or reverse progression of the disease itself or provide a cure. The goal is to prevent and relieve suffering and to improve quality of life for people facing serious, complex illness. Very often palliative care is taken to refer to alleviating the effects of cancer, but it does refer to any progressive illness such as progressive pulmonary disorders, renal disease, chronic heart failure, and progressive neurological conditions.

The reason for presenting pain associated with palliative care as distinct from acute or chronic pain is that palliative care often contains elements of both. Patients may experience acute pain during the investigative or surgical treatment elements of their disease journey. Indeed acute pain of unexplained origin may be the trigger that encourages patients to seek medical help in the first instance. Later on patients may well be subjected to chronic pain as their disease progresses

How can pain associated with palliative care be managed? The pain associated with palliative care is multifactorial and complex, consisting of pain associated with the disease and pain associated with the disease treatment. The World Health Organisation (WHO) analgesic ladder provides a stepwise framework for the pharmacological management of pain (see *Figure 1*).

- Step 1 — non-opioid drugs are the first line of analgesia. They usually control mild pain and where necessary may be supplemented with other drugs. Non-opioids are often underestimated as analgesics and there is a tendency to forget how useful they can be. The sort of drugs you may see prescribed at this stage includes paracetamol and non-steroidal anti-inflammatory drugs (NSAIDS) such as ibuprofen

- Step 2 — if the regimen employed in step one fails to control pain, or the patient reports increasing pain, then the second line of analgesic therapy is to move to a weak opioid. This weak opioid may be given with the non-opioid or used to completely replace the non-opioid drug; a commonly used example of this is paracetamol and codeine. Again, other drugs may be used if necessary. Bear in mind that the other medications may include laxatives to overcome opioid induced constipation as well as other analgesic drugs

- Step 3 — continuing pain demands the use of a strong opioid. The drug of choice in the UK is generally morphine.

Although the WHO analgesic ladder is seen as a stepwise progression the important thing is making sure that the patient is commenced on the ladder at the right level for them. Some patients will need to be started on a pain management regime that equates to step 3, whilst other will enter the ladder at step 1.

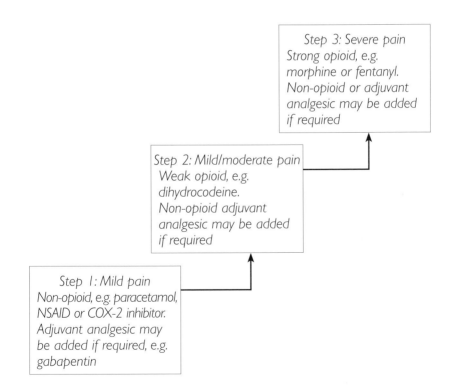

Figure 1. World Health Organisation analgesic ladder.

Pain assessment

Although there are many methods of assessing pain, some of which will be outlined within this section, there are five important rules to be remembered, regardless of the assessment method used:

1. Pain should be assessed regularly
2. The person best placed to comment on the patient's pain is the patient
3. The results of pain assessments should always be recorded
4. The results of pain assessments should always be acted upon
5. The patient should always be believed.

These rules could be expressed as Assess, Involve (the patient), Record, Act, Believe. Increasingly the responsibility for pain assessment is being seen as a part of the role of non-registered healthcare providers and an important part of that assessment is the obligation that rests upon the person undertaking the pain assessment to ensure that appropriate action is taken. Whilst healthcare assistants are not able to administer medications or to request medication review, they should understand that they have a duty to ensure that their assessment of a patient's pain is acted upon by those members of the team who can prescribe the adequate medication.

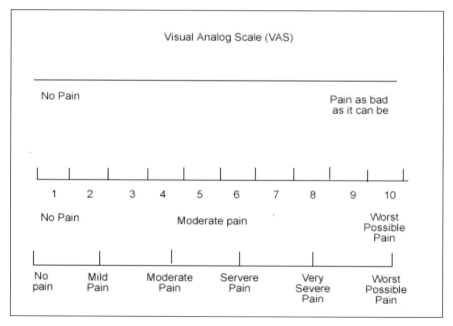

Figure 1. Examples of visual analogue scales.

Assessing acute pain

If pain is to be managed appropriately and to the satisfaction of the patient it should be assessed on a regular basis. A good pain assessment is more than just asking the patient: '*Do you have any pain?*' The assessment should include the use of a recognised measurement tool and formal and accurate documentation.

Commonly used acute pain assessment tools include visual analogue scales (VAS). Sometimes referred to a pain thermometers, a VAS consist of a 100mm line, either vertical or horizontal with either verbal descriptions or numbers from 1–10 (see *Figure 1*). Patients are asked to describe, mark or 'score' their pain at 2–4 hourly intervals or within 20 minutes of being given analgesia.

Other assessments use a 0–3 scale where 0 is no pain, 1 is mild pain, 2 is moderate pain and 3 is severe pain. The difficulty with this approach is that it is sometimes difficult for patients to decide whether their pain is mild or moderate. Also, with both types of pain assessment tool patients will often hesitate to describe their pain as 'severe' or rate it as '10' preferring to keep something in reserve in case the pain gets worse. It should be made clear to patients that they should make full use of all the choices the assessment tool provide them if their pain is to be managed appropriately.

Sometimes, healthcare practitioners are reluctant to believe a patient's report of pain, especially if the patient concerned has been sleeping, leaving the ward area to smoke or even sitting quietly watching television. The feeling is that if they can do those things they cannot possibly be in the amount of pain they say. This is a dangerous and unprofessional assumption as any one of those activities may help to act as a distraction for the patient helping them to cope with their pain and cannot be taken as proof that the patient is over-estimating the amount of discomfort they are in.

Assessing chronic pain

It has already been emphasised that pain is more than simply a physical reaction to stimuli. In acute pain the patient's fear or anxiety may contribute to how they perceive their pain severity and such factors play an integral part in the care of the chronic pain patient. It is sometimes difficult for such patients to get taken seriously by the medical, nursing and social care professionals who, if there is no clear organic cause for the pain, may imply that the patient is faking their symptoms for reasons of their own, to obtain benefits for example, or assume that the root cause of the patients behaviour is psychological in origin. Therefore chronic pain patients tend to get depressed, anxious, demanding and angry, which can make them a challenge.

Given the extremely complex nature of the chronic pain experience the assessment of pain that is appropriate for such patients must be in more depth than the assessments used for the acute pain patients.

Asking patients to keep a pain diary can also be useful in providing clues to activities that help or hinder living with a chronic pain problem. Such a strategy can also help to make the sufferer feel that they are working in partnership with their health carers to manage their pain.

Assessing pain associated with palliative care

It has already been established that pain associated with palliative care is a complex phenomenon. Pre-existing painful conditions do not disappear when a progressive disease is diagnosed. Therefore when assessing such pain it is important that the carer differentiates between the different sources of pain that such patients may experience (see *Table 1*).

It can be seen from *Table 1* that the numerous causes of pain that potentially impact upon such individuals means that numerous medication may be required. A patient who requires WHO analgesic ladder step 3 analgesia for the management of their cancer may still need the NSAIDs they are accustomed to take for their arthritis. The healthcare assistant, being the person who spends care-giving time with the patient, can be instrumental in ensuring that nursing and medical staff are aware of previous medication history.

Providing comfort

Healthcare assistants have a significant role to play in the pain management of their patients. Although they do not have the responsibility for the administration of medication there are a number of strategies they can implement whilst waiting for pharmacological responses to materialise. For the purpose of this section of the chapter we will divide comfort provision into physical, psychological and spiritual comfort and explore the contribution of the healthcare assistant through a number of exemplar case studies.

Table 1.	Cause of pain in the palliative care patient
Cause	**Example**
Pain caused by the progressive disease	Tumour infiltration of surrounding tissue
Pain caused by treatment	Neuropathic pain from chemo-therapy-induced nerve damage
Pain caused by disease associated debility	Pressure sores
Pain unrelated to the disease or its treatment	Migraine, arthritis

Physical comfort

If you think about a time when you had a small stone in your shoe, you will recall how very uncomfortable and painful it can become in a very short period of time. It is surprising how much small physical discomforts can contribute to the distress of the patient. Such issues are often very easy to address but can provide immeasurable comfort to the patient.

Case study 1

Emily is 84, and has a hip fracture; she is unfit for surgery and is confined to her bed. She has breathing problems and is on oxygen. On assessment she complains that her pain score is 7 on a 10 point visual analogue scale. How can the healthcare assistant make Emily comfortable whilst waiting for her pain relief to be administered?

In this case study, Emily has a number of problems, the resolution of which is within the remit of the healthcare assistant. As an older person Emily is likely to have fragile skin so it is important to take extra care when handling her. In addition to regular examination of pressure points and sores, using hand lotion and providing a simple hand massage can be both therapeutic and soothing. Oxygen therapy tends to dry patients' mouth and a lip balm could help relieve the discomfort of dry lips. If the inside of the mouth seems dry, giving ice chips or sips of iced water will also help. These are simple actions but will provide a great deal of ease for the patient. Likewise, hospitals tend to be overheated institutions which can lead to dryness around the lips and eyes and a damp cloth placed over closed eyes might relieve dryness. Sitting or lying in one position puts constant pressure on sensitive skin, which can lead to painful bed sores (sometimes called pressure ulcers). Turning the person from side to back and to the other side every few hours may help prevent these. If patients are trying to move themselves in their beds elbows and heels are prime sites to become sore very quickly and should have special attention. However another reason to help your patients to move is to help to make them comfortable in their bed or chair. Sometimes the pain associated with stiffness or being in one position for a long period of time can be quickly relieved by a simple change of position. This is particularly noticeable for a patient like Emily who may be experiencing severe discomfort because they are short of breath and helping them to sit in the position that is the most comfortable for them and helps to ease their breathing is as important a pain relieving measure as the provision of analgesia.

The case study cited above has shown how, with some imagination and empathy, the healthcare assistant can use physical comfort measures as adjuncts to pharmacological pain relieving strategies.

Psychological comfort

Ferrell (1996) suggests that nurses provide psychological comfort through supporting patients in sustaining their own coping resources. As the healthcare assistant is often the person who not only spends the most time at the bedside but also may have a special rapport with the patient, awareness of how to provide psychological comfort is important. Psychological issues play a part in the reporting of pain and simple provision of psychological comfort can enhance the effect of painkillers.

Case study 2

Dave is 16 years old and presents with severed tendons in his hand after punching through a plate glass window. He sustained his injury during a drunken night out whilst celebrating his brother's stag do. He is tattooed and heavily pierced, and presents as very aggressive and demanding. He is scheduled for emergency surgery but he has been a problem patient since admission, swearing and shouting and demanding increasingly large doses of painkillers and reporting no effect from the analgesia he has been given. He has made himself extremely unpopular with the staff and none of them go into his single room unless they really have to. None of his friends had come in with him. His mother is on her way but has not yet arrived.

What psychological comfort could the healthcare assistant offer in this scenario?

Patients such as Dave can present a challenge for nursing staff. Stockwell (1972) has highlighted how the 'unpopular patient' can be treated poorly by healthcare staff, and Johnson (1997) has emphasised how nurses use social judgment to make assumptions about their patients appearance and behaviour and further explored how these judgement affect the care provided.

This is a young man who is in an unfamiliar situation. He is probably scared, worried about his parent's reaction to his predicament and striving to get attention and support from nursing staff who are not willing to engage with him. His demands for pain relief and his overestimation of his pain score all point to a patient who is in psychological discomfort. In this situation the best thing that a healthcare assistant can do is spend some time listening to the patient, reassuring him by explaining how the unfamiliar world in which he has found himself operates, and providing him with what Ferrell (1996) refers to as 'anticipatory guidance' — that is charting his future care expectation and situations may provide the patient with the psychological resources he needs in order to cope. This may involve a negotiation on behaviour, the provision of information to a level that the patient dictates, and allowing privacy to express emotion. Helping the patient to focus upon the strengths and competences they have to manage the situation can also help.

Spiritual comfort

Spiritual care is often used as a synonym for religious care. For example, facilitating a Muslim patient with prayers or ensuring that the appropriate religious practitioner is available when the patient requests them does contribute to the provision of spiritual comfort. However this is not always the case. It is perfectly possible to have a spiritual dimension to one's life without necessarily subscribing to an orthodox or organised religion. A broad definition that will be used in this section is that:

> *'Spiritual care is person-centred care which, through affirmation, enables a person to make the best use of all their personal and spiritual resources in facing and coping with the doubts, anxieties and questions which arise in a health care setting and often accompany ill health and suffering.*
>
> NHS Education for Scotland (2008)

This generic definition can be seen to focus upon the human spirit rather than upon any particular religious belief, and this is probably the area of spirituality upon which the healthcare practitioner is advised to focus. However taking such a generic stance to spiritual comfort can mean that the novice healthcare assistant may find it difficult recognise situations when the provision of such care is appropriate. Work carried out by Haigh and Johnson in 2007 with 74 health care educators from 19 different countries identified five broad themes that could be used to categorise spiritual care (*Table 2*). These themes (use of self, prayer, end of life, bereavement and facilitation of religious practice), and the examples that are used to illustrate them, help to indicate the situation in which spiritual comfort is important. The interesting thing about the examples contained within *Table 2* is that they do not require special training or specific professional qualifications; they are simple manifestations of human caring in stressful situations. The willingness and courage to use yourself in the delivery of spiritual comfort is one that can be developed as your experience in healthcare settings increases.

Table 2.	Examples of provision of spiritual comfort
Theme	**Examples of spiritual care**
Use of self	• Therapeutic touch to reduce pain • Being there with patients
Prayer	• Praying with the family of a dying patient with their permission • Remaining quietly with the patient during prayer • Maintaining eye contact
End of life	• Discussing end of life issues with a patient and family including beliefs and values in order to help them clarify their spiritual needs • Talking with patient about their diagnosis
Religious/spiritual	• Baptising a baby who is likely to die • Repositioning the bed of Muslim patients who may prefer to face Mecca to pray • Supportive counselling • Allowing personal spiritual needs of the clients to be met
Bereavement	• Supporting a family when a baby dies • Comforting grieving family members who have just lost their child

The provision of spiritual comfort is a key component in the management of spiritual pain in much the same way that pain-relieving drugs are key components in the management of acute pain, as is allowing the patient to express their fear and anger in a safe and no-judgemental environment. However there is equally a case to be made for agreeing with the patient if they feel their situation is unfair or for facilitating access to spiritual help from clergy or community leaders if requested.

Conclusion

An understanding of the specific types of medication that can be used is something that is the primary concern of registered care staff, however issues such as assessment and acting upon patient self-reports of pain are the responsibility of any individual who comes into contact with a person in pain, regardless of its cause. The application of comfort-focused care can go some way towards the relief and management of all types of pain.

For healthcare assistants, it is recognised that dependence upon qualified nurses to deliver analgesia can be a professional frustration, however this chapter has outlined some strategies available to the non-registered carers for the provision of pain relief and comfort which can help to alleviate patient discomfort and promote full participation in the management of pain.

Carr E, Mann E (2000) *Pain. Creative approaches to effective management*. Macmillan Press, London

Ferrell BR, McCaffery M, Rhiner M (1992) Pain and addiction: an urgent need for change in nurse education. *Journal of Pain and Symptom Management* **7**: 141 8

Ferrell B (1996) *Suffering*. Jones & Bartlett Publishers

Haigh C, Johnson M (2007) Attitudes and Values of Nurse Educators: An International Survey. *International Journal of Nursing Education Scholarship* **4**(1):

International Association for the Study of Pain (1986) Classification of chronic pain. Descriptions of chronic pain syndromes and definitions of pain terms. *Pain* S1–S226

Johnson M (1997) Nursing power and Social Judgement. Ashgate

NHS education for Scotland (2008) Spiritual Care. Available from http://www.nes.scot.nhs.uk/spiritualcare/ (accessed 13/10/08)

McCaffery M, Beebe (1994) *Pain: A clinical manual of nursing practice*. Mosby. London

Stockwell F (1972) *The Unpopular Patient*. RCN Publications

CHAPTER 11

Caring for sick children

Angela Grainger

There are many differences between caring for adults and caring for children and therefore different skills are required. The medical speciality of children's illness is known as paediatrics, and the aim of this chapter is to give you an oversight of the particular skills healthcare assistants working in a paediatric setting need, and why these are important. This chapter mainly covers the needs of children in hospital but the key principles equally apply to nursing children in their own home or a community setting. In fact, sick children and those who have continuing care needs are wherever possible cared for in their own home because emotionally this is better for the child and the family. As sick children's nursing requires specific skills hospitals and primary care trusts employ nurses especially trained for the role. These are nurses registered with the Nursing & Midwifery Council (NMC) and have the designation of Registered Sick Children's Nurse, or Registered Nurse Child Health.

As a healthcare assistant you are responsible to your employing organisation for the duties you undertake and the way in which you perform these. You will be working alongside and under the supervision of a registered nurse as it is the registered nurse who has the authority to diagnose the nursing needs of the patient and to draw up an appropriate plan of care to meet these needs, and to evaluate the effectiveness of the care given. Healthcare assistants, in working alongside a sick children's nurse, are enabled to understand the whole needs of the child and his or her family and to demonstrate that this is taken into account during care delivery.

Paediatric staff must be prepared to work with children who have varying degrees of sickness ranging from the not-so-sick to those who are critically ill. Seeing a very sick child who might also have horrific injuries can be a frightening experience. Sometimes it is difficult to see the child for all the life-saving equipment attached to them. Nursing children is therefore not always about cuddles and play, vital though these are, and the important thing to know about the nature of being a sick children's nurse is that it is significantly different from the work of a nursery nurse or pre-school teacher where in the main, well children are encountered.

All paediatric staff need to have a non-judgemental attitude and be approachable as you are likely to be working alongside a lot of other agencies in order to meet each child's, and therefore also the family's, needs. These agencies include state schools, specially designated schools that cater for children who have special or particular needs, specialist counsellors, and social services.

In the event of a particularly horrible set of circumstances the employing organisation can arrange debriefing and counselling sessions for the staff involved. Staff can also support each other by undertaking group reflective practice sessions. Time can then be taken to see what went well in handling a certain situation so that staff agree to use the same tactics again, or alternatively what did not go quite so well. Staff can then agree on how any future similar event will be handled more appropriately. Reflective practice sessions are not just for the registered staff: healthcare assistants often have a lot to contribute to these as they are the front-line staff who have regular direct patient contact and who therefore see things from this perspective.

The child's behaviour

Whilst it is essential that all who work with children in whatever capacity should have a genuine liking of children and a concern for their welfare, this is not of itself sufficient to guarantee that the nursing needs of a sick child will be identified and met.

Sick children often regress in behaviour and might behave much younger than their years. They might therefore be both physically and emotionally demanding throughout each 24-hour period, and if the attending adult is neither prepared for this nor trained to understand and to respond appropriately it can lead to a fraught situation. Sick children are ill children, not naughty ones, although you will see temper tantrums and other expressions of anger and upset. Understanding why a child is behaving in a certain way, either physiologically or psychologically, is the essential starting point for any care plan and which obviously includes the plan of medical treatment.

Babies and young children respond to their feelings. They have not yet learned how to rationalise in a logical adult sense so they do not have a mature interpretive understanding of what is happening to them and how their emotional responses are associated with events. They cannot therefore make an adult judgement on whether they are over-reacting and that a change in behaviour is required.

The rational logic of a child depends on the child's age, intellectual development, and the overall type of environment in which they nurtured. All babies and children have their own personalities, which are still in the process of being developed. Paradoxically though sick children might emotionally need more physical comforting in the form of cuddles or gentle face stroking they might, on occasions, resist or resent it. This can be frustrating and upsetting to those in attendance on the child as very often you feel you want to give physical comfort, but you cannot impose your will on the child. There are occasions when gentle restraint is required, such as wrapping a child up in a blanket so that both arms and legs are encased in the blanket to prevent kicking out whilst a particular procedure is undertaken. This has to be done in a caring manner and for a known and accepted reason which has been explained to the parent(s) in advance and their permission obtained. The registered nurse will take the lead on this. We must not usurp or undermine the position of the parents, close family or legal guardian.

A degree of emotional maturity is required for nursing sick children as it is their needs that must be met, or adapted to, and not those of the attending healthcare professional. Unless it is an emergency or urgent situation where life or limb is endangered, paediatric staff must be flexible in their overall approach when interacting with the child and with the parents. Nursing sick children in a non-emergency situation is not for those who like to give care in a very structured, time-organised way.

Very young children do not understand the concept of time therefore, for example, taking of a 4-hourly temperature at set times means nothing to them. The child might be busily engaged in a play activity and not want to be interrupted. You often have to coax and cajole children to co-operate in order to avoid any unnecessary upset or trauma for the child. This is not the same as 'spoiling' the hospitalised child. Everything around the child will be different from what he or she is used to. There are lots of strangers, strange smells, sight and activities, and strange noises. The child's normal routine which helps to give an inner sense of safety and security has been altered by circumstances beyond the child's control. From the child's perspective it is natural that he or she might feel traumatised by being transported to such an environment.

The child should be given time to get to know his or her new surroundings. If another child can be heard crying or making distressed noises then the child being admitted, or who is about to be examined, may become apprehensive and fearful. This can make co-operation problematic. Even in an emergency situation when several senior registered healthcare professionals are attending to the child it is important to still talk to the child reassuringly, and often it is the healthcare assistant who will comfort and support the parents through this distressing and traumatic time.

Playing

If the child is admitted for an elective surgical procedure and feels quite well there could be a bewildered resentment stemming from a lack of understanding as to why the procedure is necessary. If the hospitalisation is the result of an emergency situation, and particularly where recovery is likely to be protracted and the illness/injury is associated with pain and discomfort, the child can think this is a punishment for being an unworthy or naughty child. Play activity is not therefore just time-filling. For a child, play equates with an adult's working time, and when children are well and have the energy for active play you can see how hard they work at it. It is through play that children acquire further knowledge of the world and learn new skills. When children are experiencing a strange or upsetting situation they need a way of coming to terms with what is happening and need to be helped to find ways of coping. Play is therefore also cathartic. For children who have difficulties expressing themselves play can be diagnostic if the play activity is designed to uncover their innermost feelings about what it is that is worrying or alarming them. Play therapists are the experts in this area and many hospitals employ them. Healthcare assistants working in child health should seek an opportunity to spend time with the play therapist to gain further insight into the role and how it helps children, not least because healthcare assistants are often the ones playing with the children.

Other key skills that those working with children need to have are patience, gentleness, and the ability to see things through the eyes of the child. By understanding the child's perspective we are able to communicate with the child much more meaningfully. Involving the parent(s) by letting the child sit on mother or father's lap for a physical examination, or by letting a parent apply the temperature measuring strip to the child's forehead, or in the armpit, and to make a game out of this, perhaps even allowing the child to take the parent's temperature, often helps to forge a relationship between the child and the attending healthcare professional. Knowing how to play, and possessing a lively imagination is another skill paediatric staff need to have. Often a teddy or a doll, or even a piece of cloth that is the child's personal comforter and which has been given a name by the child and therefore has a personality, even if to the adult eye it is an inanimate object, has to be 'examined' ahead of or alongside the child as this gives the child confidence.

Family centred care

To give holistic care to children we need to remember that the child is part of a societal setting which makes up the lived experience of the child's world. This means that in addition to meeting the child's needs you have to consider those of the immediate family which includes parents, siblings (brothers and sisters), and grandparents, and also close childhood or school friends who might regularly visit. The most important thing to remember is that each child does not come in isolation.

Smith et al. (2002) explain that in paediatric nursing the nurse needs to know how to work with the family in caring for the child. It is important to understand the particular structure of each child's family.

What is family?

It is important to remember that each child's family may not mirror-reflect your own experience of family, or of what you expect a family to look like or how you would expect a family to behave. There are many variations of what is considered a normal family, therefore a family can be said to consist of any stable unit in which the child is being brought up. The family is considered to be a kinship grouping of adults, or adults and children, who may not necessarily share the same residence. Some children will have a mother and father living together, whilst some will have equal access and contact to their parents although the parents live apart. Some children will be in a single parent family, and some will be with same-sex parents. Other children will not be with their parents but will be living with foster parents or in a care home facility. The UK does not have a legal definition of the family as such, but the UK is a ratified signatory of both the International Covenant on Civil and Political Rights (1966), which guarantees the right of 'the family' to be protected, and the United Nations (UN) Convention on the Rights of the Child (1991). The UN, whilst not giving a strict definition of the family, states that it is:

> '...convinced that the family, as the fundamental group of society and the natural environment for the growth and well-being of all its members and particularly children, should be afforded the necessary protection and assistance so that it [the family] can fully assume its responsibilities within the community.'
>
> United Nations (1990: 1)

Whatever the make-up of the child's family and how this might look to those outside that group, those in it are the people who are important to the child and therefore they are the ones with whom the members of the healthcare team need to establish a rapport and a working relationship.

Meeting children's needs

The UN also states that:

> '...the child should be fully prepared to live an individual life in society, and brought up in the spirit of the ideals proclaimed in the Charter of the United Nations, and in particular in the spirit of peace, dignity, tolerance, freedom, equality and solidarity.'
>
> United Nations (1990: 1)

It is from these generally accepted rights that *Every Child Matters* (DH, 2004) was developed in an effort to ensure that children were recognised as individuals in their own right and with their own specialised needs. As part of these rights it is recognised that children have the right to be cared for by people who have the appropriate specialised knowledge, skills, and personal motivation and commitment to do so.

This is not a new idea. In 1959 the *Platt Report* (Ministry of Health, 1959) recommended that sick children should be looked after by registered nurses specially trained for this role and that children should be cared for in an appropriate child-friendly environment, meaning children's hospital wards. The *Platt Report* also stated that parents, particularly mothers where young children are concerned, had the right to stay with the child when in hospital. Surprising as it may seem at the time of the *Platt Report* many children were cared for on adult wards, by nurses trained to work with adult patients, and parents were rarely allowed to visit. However, research undertaken by Bowlby (1965) showed that children need to be with people they know and with whom they have close ties if they are to cope with stressful situations. Enforced separation is emotionally damaging to children and has long term implications on the child's future abilities to establish and maintain positive emotional relationships. From Bowlby's work a pressure group, The National Association for the Welfare of Children in Hospital (NAWCH) was established and this campaigned for the rights of children to have their mothers and fathers with them in hospital. NAWCH is now called Action for Sick Children and the organisation continues to work for the rights of children and their parents in the event of children being hospitalised.

Healthcare assistants have an important role in this relationship as they are frequently one of the first people that the child and family meet when they arrive on the ward or in the clinic. First impressions are extremely important in order gaining the trust and confidence of the child and the parent(s). How the child is received on the ward or in the clinic influences the perception of the child and the parent(s) on the whole treatment experience. If a child sees that the healthcare professionals are developing a positive rapport with the parents and that the parents are warming to that interaction and that trust is being established then the child will follow the lead of the parents and become more relaxed.

Siblings and young close school friends who visit may also need a comforting, listening ear. They often need reassurance that the child will get well and that hospitalisation is not something every child has to undergo. If the child's injuries were sustained as a result of a genuine accident but in the course of normal playing then the other children involved can feel guilty and be quite traumatised. If the child has a life-limiting illness then the siblings need to be helped to understand what is happening and to be helped to cope with a normal grieving process. Even in sad situations a conscious child needs to have regular contact with close family. For a child whose condition necessitates being nursed in isolation a telephone inside the isolation room can mean 'telephone cuddles' rather than just telephone conversations (Grainger, 2008). From the point of view of a parent who is rooming in with a child, this telephone link with the outside world can feel like a lifeline.

Grandparents often help out in the care of other children, and also comfort their own children, the parents, at this distressing time. Healthcare assistant can often spend time with grandparents providing cups of tea and emotional support. Grandparents experience a double blow when a grandchild is terminally ill; they are coping with losing a beloved grandchild and also have to see in close-up how their own child, the mother or father of the ill child, is having to come to terms with losing their own child.

Communication

Good communication is a fundamental skill in nursing. Communication with the parents/career's is important but we must also be able to talk appropriately to each individual child. Wherever possible the child should be included in the conversation. They should be spoken to using age-appropriate language; in this way even a very small child can be included in the conversation.

Babies who have no hearing problems are soothed by the tone of a gentle voice, and if you are to care for a baby regularly then the baby will become familiar with your voice.

An adolescent would expect to be given the opportunity to lead some aspects of the conversation. This helps to make the child feel included in the process and that they have some choice in what is happening to them. Equally, the best person to tell you how the child is feeling and how much pain or discomfort they are in, is the child. Remember, everything we do is about keeping the child at the centre of the care.

Essential things to cover in paediatric communication includes:

- What name does the child like to be called? Is this a pet name or his/her actual first name?
- Mothers may have a different surname to that of the child. It is important to establish this for safe documentation and record-keeping. For continuity of care, and to ensure our obligations are met in relation to the safeguarding of children, where a child might have multiple emergency department attendances or admissions to different hospitals across the country, check to see if the child has been known to have a different

surname or family name to the one being used now
- What does the child like to eat and drink? Are there any special dietary needs in order to avoid any allergic reactions, for example a lactose intolerance? Does the child need a particular diet in relation to a known diagnosis, for example being a diabetic (glucose control)? Are there any cultural dietary requirements such as being a vegetarian, or needing halal meat, etc?
- What word(s) does the child use for going to the toilet? It is important to know this so the child's toiletry needs are met swiftly and therefore the child's dignity is maintained. Children who are continent and potty trained get very upset if they have a toileting accident because no-one understands what they are saying. If the child is being potty trained has the parent(s) brought the child's own potty? If not, see if it is possible to have this brought in because otherwise the potty training regime might be interrupted if the child has to get to know a new and unfamiliar potty. As we have noted previously, children can regress in behaviour when in hospital so the risk of having a toileting accident is increased. As young children tend to take pride regarding potty use it is rather unkind to them to make life more difficult in this respect than it need be
- Does the child have any known allergies, for example to penicillin, latex, etc? If the child is allergic to latex you will need to use an identification wrist/ankle bands, and if the child uses nappies then the ones that have no plastic backing or sticky closure ties will need to be used
- Does the child have any phobias, for example fear of the dark, needles, etc? How is this usually handled?
- Does the child have a special toy or cuddly and is this with the child? If not, how can this be obtained? In the meantime try to offer a suitable alternative from the ward stock toys
- Will a parent(s) be staying with the child or visiting regularly and for long periods? If the child is in a single parent family ascertain if the other parent has authorised access to the child and visiting rights. Who else might be visiting, for example, siblings, grandparents, or next door neighbours? It is important to know this because whilst the child is in hospital the staff have a duty of care to know where that child is at any one time. There have been attempted snatches of children from hospital by estranged parental partners so you need to be vigilant. Also make sure you know hot to contact the parent(s) should you need to
- Has the child been in hospital before, and if so how was that experience for the child? This information allows us to build on previous positive experiences and to be alert to any factors that made it a bad experience from the child's perspective so that we can avoid or alter these if possible

- Does the child know why he or she is attending hospital or is being admitted? What has the child actually been told and by whom? Does this seem adequate from the child's conversation about this?
- Does the parent(s) have any particular concerns? If it is not in your remit to answer any complex queries then inform the parent(s) that a registered nurse will be coming to talk with them.

As with all documentation it is important to write the responses to these questions as appropriately, clearly and legibly in the patient record and to date and sign your recording.

Remember that all the information you are given is confidential and that you only have access to this information due to the work you do and because you need to know about the child's health and social situations in order to do your job properly, i.e. on a 'need to know' basis. Confidentiality must be maintained at all times by only discussing these issues with members of the healthcare team directly involved with the care of the child. Should an adolescent tell you something that he or she does not want you to relay to the parent(s) then explain to him or her that the registered nurse needs to know of this conversation and that it would be good if the adolescent could talk privately to the registered nurse. Often adolescent patients seek advice from a healthcare professional on being sexually active and the need for contraceptive advice, about teenage pregnancy or sexually transmitted diseases, substance abuse such as alcohol, or drugs consumption. There are specially qualified staff working in these areas and the registered nurse will be able to put the enquiring adolescent in touch with the professional who is best placed to help.

Safeguarding

The safeguarding of children who are in vulnerable circumstances and who could be subject to abuse is a high priority in child welfare. All staff working with children must have an up-to-date advanced Criminal Records Bureau clearance. Your employing organisation will arrange this. It is a mandatory requirement that all healthcare staff receive safeguarding training at a level relevant to their job role, and in relation to how much direct contact they have with children. Your employing organisation will have a senior clinician or manager who is designated as the safeguarding lead and who ensures that all safeguarding issues brought to their attention are processed properly so that the required action taken to protect the child is put in place. As a healthcare assistant, if you suspect any of the following it is important that you voice your concerns to the registered nurse, or to your line manager, who will then alert the safeguarding lead:

- The child's injuries do not seem to match up to the story told of how they were obtained
- On undressing a child you notice fresh or old bruising
- You see a child being smacked hard, even if this is by the parent, or spoken to very harshly so that the child seems always to be cowed and non-communicative
- You suspect the child is being starved of food or drink,
- You suspect the child is being made to do all the housework, cooking and cleaning,
- The child is being coerced into having sex,
- The child is in a home environment where there is evidence of other forms of substance abuse.

The registered nurse, or your line manager, will alert the safeguarding lead who will come and talk to you. If you feel your concerns are not being taken seriously you can then approach the safeguarding lead direct. The important thing to remember is to put the child's welfare first. This is not breaching confidentiality. It is bringing a very important matter to the attention of the person employed in your organisation who deals with these concerns, therefore it is sharing information on a need-to-know basis. It is also important to remember that social services staff are there to work with families and to help families in need, and that they do not automatically remove the child from the parents. Accurate and timely documentation is very important in healthcare but especially when safeguarding issues are highlighted.

Understanding a child's normal developmental milestones

In order to understand the differences in child physiology it is important to know how a normal child develops so that the abnormal can be recognised. The following chart shows the expected average ages for developmental milestones. It should be remembered that it is normal for children to be ahead in some aspects and delayed in others. However if a child is noticeably and significantly lagging in one or more areas of development it is a cause for concern and should be investigated. The child's mother will be able to give a clear picture of what the child can and cannot do, but remember that your own observations will tell you a great deal (*Table 1*).

Table 1.   Developmental stages of the child

Age	Motor/sensory	Social/ understanding	Speech	Fine motor skills
Birth to 1 month	Primitive reflexes. Can suck, grasp, respond to sudden sounds.	None as yet, but this starts to be learned from birth onwards.	No speech, but uses crying and gurgling noises to communicate.	No fine motor skills as yet. Has a primitive grasp reflex. Also has a primitive walking reflex.
1–3 months	Holds head up momentarily, makes crawling movements when placed on his/her back (prone position). Can lift head for a short time when prone. Can turn from side to side., particularly in response to noises. Primitive grasp reflex is fading. Posterior fontanelle is closed.	Social smile in response to another's smile. This is the beginning of social behaviour. Eyes move in response to a light or an object.	Aware that crying usually elicits a response from adults. Has a different cry in response to different causes, e.g. hunger, a wet or dirty nappy, physical discomfort, tiredness, loneliness and wanting a cuddle.	Can momentarily hold a toy but will quickly drop it.
3 months	Lifts head from prone position for short periods. Can push him/herself up on forearms. Will turn his/her head towards sound. Has lost the primitive walking reflex. Tends to flex the knees and to have a rounded back. Still needs to be supported when held.	Smiles in response to mother's face, or other known face. Has binocular co-ordination, and can follow an object up and down and side to side.	Laughs aloud and giggles. Will make sounds when spoken to. Shows pleasure in making noises.	Holds hands up in front of him and stares at them. Plays with fingers. Can carry hand or object to mouth. Will reach out for objects within reach but does not yet have the coordination to make contact with these and grasp them.

continued...

4 months	Begins to try rolling over. Can turn from back to side. Sits with adequate support.	Recognises familiar objects. Reaches out at the sight of a dangling toy. Often places toys in the mouth.	Initiates and responds to social play by smiling. Vocalises socially by gurgling and babbling when spoken to. Takes an interest in the presence of other family members. Generally enjoys having people near him/her.	Is aware of having opposing thumb movement, can therefore do more fine hand movements but tends to hold hands open.
5 months	Sits up with less back support. Balances head. Voluntarily reaches out for objects, even those beyond his/her grasp.	Continues to learn about family members.	Vocalises displeasure by crying out when a desired object is removed.	Accepts a toy handed to him/her. Can now grasp with the whole hand.
6 months	Can sit momentarily without support if placed in a forward leaning position. Can pull him/herself up to a sitting position. Can roll over completely, i.e. from front to back. Begins to shuffle when in sitting position.	Begins to distinguish strangers from known family. Will move arms and legs energetically to display a sense of frustration. May have begun teething.	Can now make recognised sounds such as '*dada*' and '*mama*'. Continues to burble and babble rather than to make distinctive speech.	Can hold objects in one or both hands briefly. Will make banging noises with toys.

continued...

7–10 months	Is beginning to learn to sit up from a lying position. Learns to crawl and to sit steadily. Likes to play with his/her feet. From 9 months onwards will try to pull him/herself to a standing position. From this he/she will progress to walking around pieces of furniture he/she can hold on to. feet with help. By 10 months he may be walking around the furniture. Learns to crawl and sit steadily for long periods. By 10 months he does not like lying down unless sleepy.	Has become increasingly aware of strangers. Usually shows signs of anxiety and/or will cry if picked up by a stranger. Shows affection and love for family members and close friends. By 10 months responds to his/her name.	Speech continues to develop. By 10 months he has one to two words.	Manual dexterity continues to improve at varying rates. By 10 months he/she should be able to hold own bottle or drinking beaker, spoon, and toys. Will start to feed him/herself finger foods such as a biscuit or a small piece of fruit. Will play simple hand clapping games and can wave.
1 year	Can crawl well, and pulls him/herself up easily. Could be walking with some support.	Can follow and obey simple commands. Is happy to play alone.	Can say single words and understand these. Can start to put words together.	Holds a cup to drink. Starts to want to be more independent in relation to eating and drinking.

continued...

18 months	Can now walk unsupported. Begins to climb stairs and up onto furniture.	Likes to be near other children but still prefers own company. Can now usually ask for toys, drink and food. Likes to be read to and be shown pictures in a story book. Begins to recognise pictures of animals. May have started potty training.	Has use of at least 20 intelligible words.	Can turn the pages of a story book. Usually likes to play with building bricks well. Will hold a pencil and scribble.
2 years	Is able to run, climb and walk upstairs. Can open doors.	May begin to play with other children but does not yet understand the concept of sharing.	Begins to make short sentences.	Can dress him/herself in simply designed clothes, but is not yet able to fasten buttons or tie laces. Can turn the TV on and off.
3 years	Can run and jump.	Knows his/ her whole name. Can be reasoned with. Beginning to play well with other children.	Can talk in short sentences. Knows and can repeat nursery rhymes.	Usually likes to draw. Can draw circular shapes and some recognisable image figures.
4–5 years	Usually continent and can now use the toilet. Is mobile and active.	Knows many letters of the alphabet and can count up to 10 or higher.	Recites and sings.	Is starting to become more independent in thoughts and actions, and is getting ready for school.

Table adapted from Hockenberry et al (2002)

General observations to note when caring for a sick child

When meeting a child for the first time many general observations can be made without touching the child at all. Ask yourself the following questions:

- How does the child appear?
- Is the child breathing steadily? Is he/she conscious, and not bleeding profusely from anywhere? You will easily notice any of these signs
- Physically, is the child excessively small or tall for his/her age? Does the child appear to be underweight, a normal weight, or overweight?
- Does the child appear to be able to see and hear?
- If the child is of talking age, how clear is the speech and are there any speech impediments such as a lisp, or a stutter?
- Is the skin clean? Is there any evidence of scratching, or bruising? Are any rashes present? If so what does the rash look like? If a purple blotchy rash is apparent and the child looks very ill then a doctor must be summoned straight away if the child is in hospital, or an emergency ambulance called if the child is at home. This rash could have the potential to be meningitis and death from this can occur very quickly
- Is the child pale or flushed in appearance? If the child looks flushed does he/she feel hot to the touch? If the child is hot and jittery he/she may have recently had a febrile convulsion, or the body's response to a very high temperature may result in a convulsion being about to occur. A fitting child can be a frightening thing to observe but the registered nurse will be with you to guide you in what to do. You need to ensure the child's airway is clear, and that when the convulsion is occurring the child does not jerk out of the arms of the person holding the child, or if in a cot or on the floor, that the child does not hurt any limbs during the jerking or thrashing stage. The registered nurse will show you to safely reduce the child's temperature
- Does the child look jaundiced (a yellow tinge to the skin, and/or to the whites of the eyes?). Is the child skin an abnormal dusky colour, or has a purple/mauve hue, especially around the nose and lips? This indicates a problem with the oxygenation of the blood and its circulation around the body. If a dusky grey or mauve/purple colour is accompanied by difficulty in breathing then this is an emergency situation that requires the attention of a doctor
- Does the child look physically comfortable? Is the child unusually quiet and remaining still, or very restless and agitated? Not all children react to pain by crying. Pain increases the physiological process of shock whereby the blood pressure falls and circulating blood volume is either

being lost as in a haemorrhage, or is being pooled into the larger blood vessels but is not being pumped effectively around the body by the heart. Shocked patients are, if not unconscious, always quietly still and very pale, with a racing but thread-like pulse rate

- Is there evidence of any pain such as holding an arm in a protective position, or of lying with the legs drawn up or in a curled up position in order to reduce abdominal pain? An earache or a headache are signified by babies and young children by stuffing their finger into the affected ear. A headache is signified by head rolling or mild head banging against a mattress

- If the child is walking about does he/she have a normal stance and gait with no limping or dragging of the lower limbs?

- Does the child's skin tone look parched and dry? If so dehydration might have occurred. If a baby under 3 months is dehydrated the fontanelles, the soft spots on the baby's head will feel sunken and depressed.

- Has the child passed urine recently, or when was the nappy last changed and was it damp? Is there any offensive odour from the urine as this could indicate a urinary tract infection

- Has the child had a bowel motion recently and what was this like? For pre-school children who are not still being breastfed and for older children a normal bowel motion (also known as faeces or stools) is a medium brown colour, is semi-solid in consistency and is easily passed. For babies and young children being breastfed a normal stool is yellow to pale brown, is formed but is a soft consistency and again is passed easily. There should never be any blood in or around the stool. If a baby is screaming and has his/her knees pulled up toward the abdomen and a redcurrant jelly-like stool is passed this is a surgical emergency and medical assistance must be sought immediately. If the motion is difficult to pass and is hard with a dry, parched appearance then constipation might be present. A registered nurse or a doctor needs to take a full medical history to confirm this and to order an appropriate treatment. Alternatively, the child may have frequency caused by intestinal hurry in passing bowel motions with the stools being semi-liquid to pure liquid in consistency. This could be diarrhoea or might be associated with a digestive malabsorption problem especially if the stool also looks and smells fatty. If the stools are offensive in odour a bacterial, fungal, or parasitic infection could be present.

By observing and making a note of the presence or absence of these signs and symptoms the healthcare assistant is performing an important duty to the child because the early and accurate notification of these enables the doctor to order the required diagnostic tests and to also make an early diagnosis thereby ensuring that the child's recovery is optimised.

The healthcare assistant is often involved in ensuring fundamental aspects of care are carried out. In relation to a child's bodily functions such care could include maintaining a safe environment, specimen collection, bathing and personal hygiene, recording clinical observations, and helping the child to eat and drink. As part of your continuing development you will be shown how to become competent in the practical aspects of children's nursing in your own clinical area where your registered nurse colleagues will act as mentors and supervisors. However, there are some general guiding principles in relation to these aspects of care and these will be outlined here.

Maintaining a child-friendly safe environment

Remember the need to comply with the Health and Safety at Work Act 1974, and as children are usually active check everything at ground level. Make sure the floor lining is not split and sticking up so that trips and falls can occur. Mop up any spillages as these occur to avoid slips and falls.

Do not let the children run around in bare feet in case a sharp object has dropped on the floor leading to injury. Do not keep the sharps bins on or near the floor; these are brightly coloured and are therefore attractive to children who will put their hands in the top and pull out a dirty needle to play with. Check all toys for any sharp edges that could cause injury. Ensure that children are appropriately supervised in the bath/shower room so that accidents such as slipping, drowning or scalding are avoided. Ensure that a baby's bath water is not so hot that it will redden and scald the skin. Add the hot water into a cold bath whilst leaving your elbow in the water to test the temperature. It should feel slightly warmer than lukewarm. Lower the baby gently and slowly into the water and observe to see if any reddening of the skin occurs. If it does, bring the baby out of the water immediately. If the baby is scalded medical attention must be sought straightaway.

Do not let the baby sit near the tap end of the bath as hot water could drip out onto the baby. Hold the baby securely. Soap the baby in the water with one hand so that your other hand is still holding the baby steady in the bath. Never leave a baby alone in the bath. Dry the baby thoroughly so there is no chapped skin. Bath time is usually a happy time for babies and young children as they love playing with water so do allow time for this.

Positioning of babies
Babies should be laid on their back in a cot. To help make small babies feel more secure and safe roll two clean towels up in a cross style and place these in a pillow case. This makes a cradle nest for the baby to lie in the midst of

and prevents them from rolling around in a large cot. Never leave a baby, or a small child, in a cot with the cot sides down in case they either roll or climb out.

Eating and drinking

If a baby is being breastfed you must assure the mother of complete privacy whilst this is being done. The mother will tell you if the baby is not latching on properly or does not seem interested in suckling. The baby's weight recordings will show whether sufficient intake is being obtained, as well as the baby's overall condition, along with the analysis of any blood tests taken. The healthcare assistant should record on the feed chart, or the fluid balance chart, that the baby was breastfed and state the time.

If a baby is being bottle fed then the bottle feed will be made up in sterile conditions in a hospital milk kitchen. Sometimes a special dietary milk formula prescribed by a doctor is ordered. The amount of milk per bottle for each individual baby is calculated on a millilitre by weight formula. If you are preparing a baby's bottle at home in the community then be sure to prepare this in accordance with strict hygiene procedures, and you must have the use of sterilising agents for bottles before use. Babies are vulnerable to gastroenteritis leading to dehydration, and poor bottle preparations are a common cause of this. Again, the healthcare assistant should note how much the baby has taken from the total amount in the bottle and record this on the feed chart. If the healthcare assistant is feeding the baby then check to see if the baby needs a nappy change beforehand, and also record any clinical observations that are due to be taken. The warmth of the feed will raise the baby's temperature, and the activity of sucking on the teat will temporarily raise the baby's pulse, which is why the clinical observations should be recorded before the baby is fed. Check that the bottle is warmed to a suitable temperature and is not so hot that it will scald the baby's mouth. Shaking a few drops onto the back of your hand is a good test of temperature. Position yourself comfortably in a chair and the baby comfortably in your arms. If the baby is not comfortable he or she will let you know. You can talk to the baby whilst the baby is sucking as this will not interfere with the taking of the feed and the baby will find this comforting. Gently rub the baby's back to help bring up any wind either halfway through the feed or at the end of the feed, whichever seems to suit the baby best. Record the feed on the feed chart and tidy up the area around the cot.

Young children may need feeding or assistance with feeding. Ensure they have been to the toilet and been supervised in washing their hands. Ensure they have a suitable height of chair so they can reach the table easily. Ensure that the food is attractively presented on the plate and that the child also has a suitable drink. Young children may need to wear a bib to catch food spillage. Make sure this is clean before you put it on the child as a dirty bib can harbour germs. For children who can feed themselves let them talk, and interact with their peers at the table as eating is a social occasion. For children who need feeding, sit either next to them or in front of them and offer a selected mixed sample of all the food on the plate in an appropriately spoon-sized mouthful. Wait until the child has finished chewing and has swallowed before offering another spoonful. Praise the child for the effort made. Do not allow mealtimes to turn into a battle of wills and learn the art of negotiation and compromise over what is ingested.

Privacy and dignity

Babies, children and young people are as entitled to having their right of privacy and dignity respected as are adults. Perform any procedures in a quiet place so that privacy is maintained. In line with safeguarding procedures, paediatric healthcare professionals should be accompanied by a parent or a colleague acting as a chaperone who may interact with the child for distraction purposes when any intimate procedure is being performed. This includes changing nappies and bathing. Wherever possible allow the mother to give continued fundamental care to her child. Ensure that the checking of nappies and changing occurs regularly and that nappies are changed as soon as the baby has used the nappy to prevent nappy rashes and to maintain the general health of the skin. Show the mother the system for the safe, hygienic disposal of nappies and the procedure for safe hand-washing. This is part of the infection control policy and is done to ensure that the risk of any infected or dirty materials cannot be passed from person-to-person resulting in outbreaks of diarrhoea and vomiting.

Specimen collection

When a urine specimen is needed a special collecting U-bag system that is adhesive to the skin (but is non-damaging to the skin) is applied over the genital area. When the baby or child urinates the urine flows into the collecting bag, which is then gently detached form the child and the urine tipped into a sterile urine pot.

If a baby or child is allergic to latex then this collection system should not be used. Instead hold the child periodically over a sterile collecting pot which is sat inside the well of a potty and catch the urine in this.

For faecal specimens a lining is placed inside the baby's nappy which allows the stool to be picked up easily by the collection spoon found inside the stool specimen pot. For older children ask them to defecate into a clean potty or bedpan and before wiping their bottom and depositing toilet paper into the potty or bedpan, spoon out the faecal specimen with the spoon provided in the special collection pot.

Remember to label accurately the specimen with the child's name, date of birth, hospital patient record number, type of specimen, and date and time collected. Remember to wear gloves for these specimen collection procedures and to wash your hands thoroughly afterwards.

Blood collection

Some experienced healthcare assistants are specially trained to take blood from children and to insert cannulae. If you are required to perform this duty you should receive proper training from a paediatric phlebotomist in accordance with the guidance and standards set by the UK Phlebotomy Association. You should only undertake this training if your job requires you to regularly take blood or to insert cannulae as otherwise your required competence will not be maintained. You should only be undertaking these competences on a solo basis after you have been signed off as competent by your phlebotomist assessor or other qualified health professional who is skilled in phlebotomy.

Remember that a local anaesthetic agent may be applied before blood being taken to stop the child from feeling the insertion of the needle; check that a sufficient area of the skin has been covered with the anaesthetic agent and that the agent has been given the required time to work as specified in the manufacturer's instructions.

Recording clinical observations

Readers are advised to also read the chapter on recording clinical observations. In babies and young children Tempa Dots, placed in the crook of the armpit, are used to record the body's temperature. Rectal temperatures are rarely if ever taken as the act of inserting the thermometer stimulates bowel movements and if the patient already has a bowel problem this can make the problem worse. Mercury thermometers are no longer used as mercury is toxic and a broken glass thermometer will leak mercury. For older children (usually from the age of 8 years) a tympanic thermometer is inserted gently into the outer eardrum. Each recording nozzle tip must be used once only and then discarded to prevent any spread of infection. The normal temperature range for babies and children is 36–37 degrees centigrade.

The normal pulse range varies according to the age of the child. Babies can have a pulse rate of around 110–160 beats per minute. For younger children it is around 100–150 beats per minute, and as the child gets older and moves into adolescence and then adulthood it settles to around 80 beats per minute. These ranges are not absolute and the overall condition of the child must be taken into account. Anyone who is nervous will have a higher pulse rate. Very sporty children will have a lower pulse rate.

Respiratory rate varies in accordance with age and overall condition. Babies have a higher respiration rate at around 40 respirations per minute, and which gradually lessens as age increases until the rate is around 15–20 respirations per minute at age 12 years and more.

The blood pressure is rather more difficult to detect in babies and young children which is why sophisticated and sensitive electronic monitoring equipment is used should the child's condition necessitate frequent blood pressure monitoring. The normal practice is to monitor the systolic pressure in millimetres of mercury (mmHg).

Crisp and Rainbow (2007) define the following blood pressure recordings per age range. For a baby the usual systolic range is 70–90 mmHg. Hypertension (high blood pressure) in babies starts from a reading of 115/75 mmHg. For children between 5 and 12 years of age the accepted systolic pressure is 90–110 mmHg. For this age group hypertension is from 125/80 mmHg. For children over 12 years of age the accepted systolic pressure is 100–120 mmHg, with hypertension being from 135/85 mmHg.

The practical competences of taking and recording clinical observations will be acquired under supervised practice in the workplace.

Conclusion

This chapter has outlined the main principles of caring for sick babies and young children so that the distress of being ill, and any fear and anxiety accompanying this is lessened by being cared for by competent and understanding paediatric staff. Another aim is the provision of practical advice to healthcare assistants who are new to working with babies and young children, or who are new to working in a paediatric setting, so that any anxieties they might have are lessened. Ultimately it is hoped that all who work with babies and children will find this a satisfying and deeply rewarding experience and that the advice offered here helps to facilitate this.

Bolby J (1965) *Child Care and the Growth of Love*. Penguin, Harmondsworth

Crisp S, Rainbow J (eds) (2007) *Emergencies in Paediatrics and Neonatology*. Oxford University Press, Oxford

DH (2004) *National Service Framework (NSF) for Children, Young People, and Maternity Services*. Department of Health, London

Grainger A (2008) Children's Nursing — principles and practicalities in caring for family and friends. Br J Health Care Assistants **3**(8): 35

Hockenberry MJ, Wilson D, Winkelstein ML, Kline NE (2002) *Wong's Nursing Care of Infants and Children*. 7th edition. Moseby, USA

Ministry of Health (1959) *The Report of the Committee on the Welfare of Children in Hospital (Platt Report).* HMSO, London

Smith L, Coleman V, Bradshaw M (2002) *Family-centred Care.* Palgrave, Hampshire

UN (1990) *Convention on the Rights of the Child.* United Nations, New York

CHAPTER 12

Common mental health problems in older adults

Catherine Bryant, Emma Ouldred

There are significant numbers of older people with mental health problems. Estimates from the Department of Health (DH) suggest that, in the UK, mental health problems are present in 40% of older people who attend their GP, in 50% of older adult in-patients in general hospitals, and in 60% of residents in care homes (DH, 2005). Sadly older people with mental health problems often do not have satisfactory support and services. Up to a third of carers also have some form of mental illness (Singleton et al, 2002).

The *UK Inquiry into Mental Health and Well-being in Later Life* (2007) made 35 recommendations to improve mental health services for older people and called for action to eliminate age discrimination, challenge stigma, ageism and defeatism, work on preventing problems, support older people and their carers to help themselves and each other, improve housing, health and social care services. The inquiry also called on the government to provide leadership and overthrow years of under-funding in older people's mental health services.

Depression is the most common mental health disorder, affecting three times as many older people as dementia. Delirium, schizophrenia, bipolar disorders, alcohol misuse, anxiety, agoraphobia and adjustment disorders make up most of the remainder (Royal College of Psychiatrists, 2008).

At any one time older adults occupy up to two thirds NHS beds and up to 60% of these patients will have mental health needs-mainly dementia, delirium and depression (Royal College of Psychiatrists, 2005).

Although this chapter focuses on the recognition and management of dementia, delirium and depression it must be remembered that there also exist poor levels of services for people growing older with long-standing mental health conditions such as schizophrenia.

Dementia

There are 683,597 people with dementia in the UK (Knapp et al, 2007). However, this figure is expected to rise to 1,735,087 by 2051. The incidence of dementia rises with age such that it affects one in 14 people over the age of 65, rising to one in six over the age of 80. However, it is not a disease exclusively of old age and there are approximately 15,000 people living in the UK with young onset dementia —onset before the age of 65 (Alzheimer's Society, 2009). People with learning disabilities such as Down's syndrome are likely to develop Alzheimer's disease at an earlier age than the general population. The average age for a person with Down's syndrome to develop dementia is 52.8 years (Janicki, 2002).

Guidance on dementia issued by the National Institute for Health and Clinical Excellence (NICE, 2006) aims to support people with dementia and their carers. This guidance sets out good principles of care in dementia including early diagnosis, access to specialist services and management of the symptoms of dementia including challenging behaviour. The guidance promotes the principle of person-centred care, meaning that all treatment and care should take into account each person's individual needs and preferences. Ideally care for a person with dementia should be based in the community with local support services that help maintain and promote their independence and wellbeing. The importance of supporting informal carers of people with dementia is emphasised and also that all health and social care staff should receive training to care for clients with dementia. Acute and general hospital trusts should plan and provide services that address the specific personal and social care needs and the mental and physical health of people with dementia who use acute hospital facilities for any reason.

The Government produced its first ever National Dementia Strategy (NDS) in February 2009. The main aims of the NDS are:

- To facilitate early diagnosis and intervention through ensuring that effective services for early diagnosis and interventions are available on a nationwide basis through the establishment of more memory clinics.

- To improve awareness of dementia through the development of a better understanding of dementia by public and professionals, and ensuring that better information is provided on how to seek help and what help and treatment is available, and tackling the stigma and misunderstandings that currently exists.

- To improve the quality of care for dementia through focusing on the improvement of liaison services that can enable effective management in hospital and intermediate care, and building better skills and understanding of dementia in the health and social care workforce so that all those working with older people develop core skills in this area.

What is dementia?

Dementia is a term used to describe the symptoms that occur when the brain is affected by specific diseases and conditions. Dementia is usually progressive and causes a loss of brain function that eventually becomes severe. Alzheimer's disease is the commonest form of dementia, as shown in *Table 1*.

Table 1.   Prevalence of dementia in the UK

Alzheimer's disease	62%
Vascular dementia/mixed dementia	27%
Dementia with Lewy bodies, fronto-temporal dementia and Parkinson's dementia	8%
Other forms of dementia such as Wernicke-Korsakoff's syndrome (alcohol related dementia), progressive supranuclear palsy, neurosyphillis, Huntingdon's disease, HIV infection and Creutzfeldt-Jacob disease	3%

Source: Knapp et al (2007)

The causes of dementia are still not fully understood. Risk factors include increasing age and injury to the brain (such as severe brain injury, stroke disease and alcohol abuse). Some forms of dementia have a genetic component. Vascular risk factors such as hypertension, diabetes and smoking are associated with Alzheimer's disease and vascular dementia are of course amenable to treatment. The main symptoms of dementia are:

- Memory loss
- Language impairment and communication problems — a decline in the ability to read, write and talk
- Disorientation — confusion over time, place and even person
- Changes in mood and/or personality
- Impaired reasoning and judgement such as reduced safety awareness (e.g. person with dementia might try and get from seat unaided even though there is a high likelihood they will fall or a person with dementia allowing a stranger into their home without knowing who they are)
- Confusion between day and night (diurnal variation)
- Apraxia — inability to perform motor tasks (e.g. difficulty performing tasks such as driving a car or in severe disease how to put on trousers)
- Agnosia — inability to recognise objects or people e.g. failure to recognise relatives)

- Behavioural disturbances such as agitation, depression, wandering and visual and auditory hallucinations.

Changes that occur in people with dementia lead to difficulties in activities of daily living such as remembering to attend hospital appointments, and reduced social functioning such as disorientation in unfamiliar environments or reluctance to interact in social activities Behavioural changes can occur such as sleep disturbance and psychological disturbance such as apathy, agitation and depression.

Main forms of dementia

Alzheimer's disease

This is the most common form of dementia seen in those aged over 65 years. During the course of the disease abnormal plaques and tangles develop within the structure of the brain, leading to the death of brain cells. This leads to a reduction of chemicals (neurotransmitters) in the brain, which affects the cell's ability to communicate with each other. Features of Alzheimer's disease include:

- Depletion of chemical messengers in the brain
- Build up of abnormal proteins: amyloid plaques, damaged nerve fibres and tau tangles (which can only be seen under a microscope)
- Medial temporal lobe (memory area of brain) is first area affected thus primary signs are often forgetfulness and confusion
- Gradual progression
- There is no cure but symptomatic relief (such as a stabilisation of symptoms or slow down in progression) may be gained from acetylcholinesterase inhibitors (e.g. donepezil, galantamine and rivastigmine)
- Computer tomography head scan may show atrophy particularly in medial temporal lobe

Vascular dementia

Vascular dementia accounts for over a quarter of all cases of dementia. It is caused by problems with the oxygen supply to the brain and diseases that contribute to vascular disease such as hypertension, diabetes and high blood cholesterol increase the risk. It is most commonly caused by a series of small strokes that individually may not cause any specific symptoms (Knapp et al, 2007). Vascular dementia and Alzheimer's disease may co-exist. This is referred to as mixed dementia. Vascular dementia affects people in different ways and thus the rate of progression will differ. However, some of the common features of vascular dementia are listed below:

- Damage to blood vessels leading to brain
- Lack of oxygen to brain causing cell death
- Symptoms may be sudden as a result of stroke
- Stepwise progression (symptoms might plateau or stabilise and then deteriorate suddenly) through a series of mild strokes
- Depression post-stroke
- Physical symptoms of stroke such as paralysis, speech impairment, incontinence
- Epileptic seizures
- Difficulty concentrating
- Hallucinations
- Delusions
- Getting lost
- Periods of acute confusion
- Computer tomography of head scan may show isolated areas of stroke damage or widespread disease of the network of small blood vessels suppling the brain.

Dementia with Lewy bodies

Lewy bodies are microscopic deposits found in damaged nerve cells. Dementia with Lewy bodies is a progressive condition where there is gradual degeneration and death of nerve cells. Its features include:

- Gradual degeneration and death of nerve cells
- Spherical protein deposits found inside damaged nerve cells: Lewy bodies
- Fluctuating cognitive levels
- Parkinsonian symptoms such as shuffling gait and tremor. Associated balance problems and increased risk of falls
- Poor concentration
- Visual hallucinations
- Neuroleptic drug sensitivity: neuroleptic (antipsychotic) drugs such as haloperidol that have been used to treat behavioural symptoms in dementia can be fatal in dementia with Lewy bodies and must be used with extreme caution
- Computer tomography scan may show mild involutional changes and atrophy.

Reversible dementia

Some dementias (mainly those due to a general medical condition) may be arrested or reversed if the condition is successfully treated before significant brain damage has occurred. Such conditions include:

- Metabolic causes such as thyroid deficiency
- Nutritional deficiency such as vitamin B12 deficiency and thiamine deficiency (often seen in malnourished people and those with alcohol problems)
- Neurological causes such as brain tumour and normal pressure hydrocephalus
- Drug toxicity such as that caused by drugs with anticholinergic activity (such as oxybutynin). Other drugs known to increase confusion include opiates such as morphine.

How the brain is affected by dementia

Dementia is usually a progressive condition associated with gradual loss of nerve cells and changes in neurotransmitters (chemical messengers that relay information between brain cells). In Alzheimer's disease for example, there is a global deterioration in brain function and eventually all areas of the brain become affected by the illness. However the pattern of deterioration differs amongst people with dementia and as such each individual may have a set of differences and experiences peculiar to them. It is useful to have a basic understanding of which parts of the brain are responsible for certain functions and to have an awareness of how changes in the brain can affect memory, thought and behaviour in people with dementia.

The brain is made up of three main sections:

- Forebrain
- Hindbrain
- Midbrain.

The hindbrain and midbrain are responsible for maintenance of basic life support functions such as blood pressure and respiration. However, the forebrain is responsible for most higher brain functions such as memory and language.

Cerebral cortex: This is the most important part of the forebrain and covers its surface. It is densely packed with brain cells. Bundles of fibres (white matter) beneath the cerebral cortex transport information around to other areas of the brain. **The lobes:** The forebrain is divided into 4 lobes: Frontal lobe (executive or management centre), parietal lobe, temporal lobe and occipital lobe. *Table 2* outlines the function of each lobe and briefly describes the kind of problems a person with dementia might experience as a result of damage to specific parts of the brain. It must also be remembered that the lobes of the brain do not function in isolation and thus damage in one area can also have an impact on other areas of brain function.

Progression of dementia

Progression of dementia may be rapid in some people but in others decline can occur gradually over a number of years. What is inevitable is that abilities will diminish over time. It might be helpful to consider classifying

Table 2.   How dementia affects brain function

	Function	**Consequence of damage**
Frontal lobe	Organising and planning actions and learning new tasks. Loss of simple movements	Inability to learn new things/follow instructions. Inability to perform simple (multi-step) tasks. People may get stuck on what they are trying to do so may do the same thing repeatedly such as unpacking/packing bags, repeatedly saying the same words
	Expression of language	Person may not know what they want to say but are unable to do so.
	Motivation centre	Person might appear lethargic and withdrawn, requiring prompting and encouragement to do things, e.g. have a wash or interact on a social level. This is often attributed to laziness. Ability to focus on tasks/solve problems might be noticed.
	Regulation of behaviour	Swearing, taking clothes off in public, inappropriate sexual activity, smearing faeces on walls, etc.
	Personality centre	Relatives might notice changes in personality such as the person with dementia not being as affectionate as they used to be, or being described as 'not the person they used to know'.

continued...

Temporal lobe	Predominantly concerned with memory. Verbal memory and the names of objects. Episodic memory: memory of events or episodes. Semantic memory: our encyclopaedia of facts enables us to remember where we put our passport, where we went to school (long-term memory). Also involved in hearing, the acquisition of memory, visual perception and ability to categorise objects.	Misplacing objects, forgetting familiar landmarks, forgetting to attend appointments or remembering birthdays, etc. Prosopagnosia, i.e. difficulties remembering faces. Difficulty understanding spoken word, forgetting recent holidays
Occipital lobe	Processing of visual information, i.e. when the optic nerve sends information from the eye to the occipital lobe it processes information to extract key information and uses it to build up a complex representation of the outside world and reveals what objects are in the environment and what they are doing	Difficulty locating objects and the environment. Problems understanding and recognising what objects are such as clothing, shower or cutlery (perceptual difficulties). Difficulty drawing objects or seeing things accurately. Problems reading and writing.
Parietal lobe	Related to information about spatial relationships and structure. Concerned with ability to put things in order or structure such as reading and writing and calculation. Related to ability to co-ordinate properly and sequence body movements. Enables us to know left from right. Receives visual information from occipital lobe and combines information into a 3D representation of what is being seen. Helps us to locate objects relative to one another such as picking something up or being able to elicit how wide a road is in order to cross safely.	Difficulty reading, writing and doing calculations. Problems dressing due to lack of coordination and associated difficulty remembering how to do something such as tying shoelaces or fastening buttons (apraxia). Perceptual disturbance such as hallucinations. Inability to differentiate between beds on a ward may mean a person with dementia may get into the wrong bed.

Adapted from Alzheimer's Society (2008), Lehr (2006), Hobson (2007) the symptoms of dementia into three stages. However, it must be remembered that not all of the features described will be present in every person and individuals may show symptoms of more than one stage at the same time. Do also note that not every person will move through each stage sequentially. Early stages of dementia include:

- Loss of short-term memory. Examples: repetitive questioning and loss of thread of conversations, missed appointments, missed collection of prescriptions
- Loss of interest in hobbies and activities. Examples: stopping attendance bridge classes or local social clubs
- Anxiety
- Difficulty handling money. Example: getting muddled up with denominations of currency
- Poor judgement. Example: impaired driving ability
- Impaired concentration
- Unwillingness to make decisions
- Difficulty adapting to change. Examples: gong on holiday
- Irritability/distress if unable to do something
- Misplacement of objects. Examples: keys, spectacles
- Readiness to blame others for 'stealing' things.

Moderate stages of dementia include:

- Increased need for support such as reminders to eat, wash, dress, and use the toilet
- Confusion regarding time and place
- Failure to recognise people and objects even though there is no impairment of sight or sense of touch (agnosia). Example: not recognising own family or reflection
- behavioural symptoms. Examples: wandering and getting lost, hallucinations (visual and auditory)
- Risky behaviour. Examples: leaving the house in night clothes, forgetting to turn taps off, leaving gas on
- Increased repetitive behaviour
- Increased forgetfulness of recent events
- Aphasia. Example: word-finding difficulty
- Apraxia (loss of ability to perform intentional movements even though the person has no paralysis, has not lost the sense of touch and knows what they are trying to do). Example: tying shoelaces
- Increased anger, upset and distress.

Advanced stages of dementia include:

- Inability to remember for even a few minutes
- Need for full assistance with washing, dressing and toileting
- Loss of ability to recognise food, self-feed and swallow effectively
- Double incontinence
- Increasing physical frailty/motor retardation — may start to shuffle or walk unsteadily, eventually becoming confined to bed or a wheelchair
- Increased risk of complications associated with prolonged immobility such as constipation, chest infection and urinary tract infections
- Increased confusion and restlessness such as searching for a dead relative
- Increased aggressive behaviour (verbal and physical)
- Disinhibition. For example: taking clothes off in public
- Night disturbance
- Uncontrolled movements, development of seizures
- Difficulty eating and sometimes swallowing
- Weight loss
- Contractures due to muscle rigidity and deconditioning
- Lack of communication including gradual loss of understanding of others.

End of life care in dementia

About 29% of people with cancer, respiratory disease or circulatory disease have dementia, and by 2010 there will be 700,000 people with dementia in their last year of life (National Council for Palliative Care, 2009). It is not inevitable that all people with dementia will reach the end stages of their disease before death. Cox and Cook (2002) describe three ways in which people with dementia die:

- People with dementia may die with a medical condition that is unrelated to the dementia, for example people in early stages of dementia who develop and subsequently die from cancer
- People with dementia may die from a complex mix of mental health and physical problems where dementia is not the primary cause of death but interacts with other conditions such as chronic obstructive pulmonary disease (COPD)
- People with dementia may die with complications associated with advanced dementia.

The development of policies and guidance specifically related to end of life care has evolved slowly, but practitioners are advised to read recent guidance published by the National Council for Palliative Care (NCPC) which explores the issues and challenges of addressing end of life care needs of people with dementia and their carers and offers practical solutions to these problems (NCPC, 2009). The National Dementia Strategy (DH, 2009) also addresses end of life care in dementia and attention is paid to this issue in the *Strategy for End of Life Care in England* recently published by the Department of Health (2008).

Management of dementia

Person-centred care
One of the main aims of management is to promote independence for the individual and maintenance of function for as long as possible underpinned by the philosophy of person-centred care (NICE, 2006). Person-centred care in dementia aims to see the person with dementia as an individual, rather than focusing on their illness and on the abilities they may have lost. Instead of treating the person as a collection of symptoms and behaviours to be controlled, person-centred care takes into account each individual's unique qualities, abilities, interests, preferences and needs (Kitwood, 1997).

Mental Capacity and the Mental Capacity Act 2005
The Mental Capacity Act 2005 came into force in 2007 and is likely to have a major impact on the way decisions are made for all practitioners working with adults who may lack mental capacity. The Act provides a statutory framework to empower people who may lack capacity to make decisions for themselves such as people with dementia. This legislation makes it clear who can take decisions, in which situations and how they should go about them. Before outlining the main clauses of the Act it is useful to consider what 'capacity' means and how capacity decisions are made. It is important to remember such decisions are situation-specific. A practitioner might consider a person does not have capacity in one area (for example managing finances) but deems a person to have capacity in another situation (such as what to wear). If a person has mental capacity (competency) they are able to make decisions for themselves. Under the terms of the Mental Capacity Act one should always assume a person has capacity unless proven otherwise. The legal definition says that someone who lacks capacity cannot do one or more of the following four things:

• Understand information given to them
• Retain that information long enough to be able to make a decision
• Weigh up the information available to make a decision
• Communicate their decision by any possible means (such as squeezing a hand or using sign language).

Psychosocial interventions in dementia

Cognitive stimulation

Current guidance recommends that people with mild to moderate dementia of all types should be offered cognitive stimulation. Cognitive stimulation can be defined as engagement in a range of activities and discussions (usually in a group) aimed at general enhancement of cognitive and social functioning (Clare and Woods, 2004). It may occur informally through recreational activities, or formally through group programmes that are designed to stimulate or engage people with dementia, or perhaps through specific training exercises designed to address specific cognitive functions. Cognitive rehabilitation programmes are usually individually tailored and target specific goals. In the care home setting this could simply mean resident discussion groups or current affairs forum.

Reality orientation

This approach is useful in the early stages of dementia when short-term memory is still relatively well preserved. It can be used to try and retain the independence of the person with dementia. However as illness progresses and short-term memory deteriorates reality orientation becomes ineffective.

The main aim of reality orientation is to help people with dementia maintain a grasp on reality (e.g. the who, what, where and how of life) and thus remain independent and able to perform activities of daily living. Reality orientation takes several forms:

24-hour reality orientation: this takes the form of a running commentary on the day and what is happening. This involves constant reiteration and reinforcement by the continual provision of verbal clues and cues which allows the person with dementia to remain aware of what it is they need to do. For example: information given by a carer might take the form of continuous dialogue while helping somebody in the morning: *'Here is your toothbrush, Mary, use it to clean your teeth like this'* [carer demonstrates action]. Miming action reminds Mary what she needs to do. This continues through the day, with carers constantly providing Mary with the clues and information to maintain her independence as much as possible.

Maintenance of routine: our lives revolve around structure and routine such as getting up, having a cup of tea, feeding the cat. Without these familiar clues and cues we too would also become disorientated. Think of how difficult people find adjusting to new routines such as retirement. A familiar routine to the day in a familiar environment is crucial in order for people with dementia to remain located in the world (Walsh, 2006). Thus an important part of reality orientation is maintenance of a familiar and structured routine and not changing a familiar environment. For example: care home residents with dementia are often much more confused when admitted to the unfamiliar environment of a hospital. This may be caused by loss of familiar landmarks, staff, change to routine and a fear of unknown.

Labelling: labelling doors, drawers, etc. with large signs or pictures enable people with dementia to be reminded of what lies within and thus helps to maintain independence. Written signs may be used first but as dementia progresses people with dementia may not recognise words and a picture might be more useful as ability to understand pictures is retained longer than that to recognise words. Carers typically label areas such as the toilet and where things should go around the house (such as the cutlery drawer). Writing an individual's name above their hospital bed may help them to adapt more quickly to new environment.

Reality orientation boards: these are basic white boards with details of place, date, weather, staff, etc. Such items help to provide a point of reference for people with dementia and reminds them of basic information which helps to orientate them. Reality orientation boards can be used in different environments including hospital wards, day centres and care homes.

Colour coding: simply colouring specific doors (such as painting all toilet doors red) can serve as useful visual prompts for people with dementia. People with dementia might wander off a ward because they are simply looking for the toilet.

Reality orientation groups: reality orientation can also take the form of special sessions whereby small groups of people meet with staff/carers on a regular basis for a fixed duration. Questions and comments are raised concerning areas such as the weather, day, date, month, history, etc. For example: a group may discuss the hot weather and then go on to reminisce about past summer holidays. It is useful to have a good knowledge of the group member's past in order to personalise the group and make subject matter more relevant.

Personal history boards and scrapbooks: history boards are pin boards placed by bedsides or a prominent place in the room of a person with dementia. Boards may contain the name of the person with dementia, photographs, mementos from the past and pictures of pets, family members and other artefacts relevant to a person's past and present. History boards are a visual point of reference for a person with dementia and a useful conversation source for carers. Personal scrapbooks are similar to history boards but are life stories collected and collated during 1:1 sessions which focus on past and present identities.

Validation therapy

Validation therapy should be regarded as complementary to reality orientation rather than a replacement (Walsh, 2006). The two therapies should be used at different stages of dementia. As dementia progresses, short-term memory will diminish to the point where it is virtually non-existent thus at this stage the clues and prompts provided by reality orientation will not be retained long enough to be useful. It becomes meaningless to reinforce our reality with regards time and place, etc. As short-term memory diminishes the long-term memory comes to the fore and people with dementia appear to be 'living in the past'. Without short-term memory the past is their reality. For example: an 80 year old person with dementia might think he is only 30 years old. He might feel he is still of working age and so it is natural for him to get up at 09.00 am and set off to 'work'. Validation therapy suggests that the obvious unreality to you should be ignored (i.e. person is 80, not 30) and you should try and understand the reality from the person's point of view. In effect you should validate the reality.

Another example of validation therapy would be the following: Bobby is aged 78 wakes up one morning at his care home and is very confused. He gets up and starts packing his bag saying he is going to meet his sister at Liverpool Station (his sister Jenny died a few years ago). Reorientating Bobby by saying Jenny has passed away will cause more upset and confusion, as will blocking his way and locking the door. Validation therapy encourages carers to talk to Bobby about his sister but maintaining the past tense. You could ask Bobby what he and Jenny used to do at Liverpool Street station and did he enjoy travelling by train. Encouraging him to talk about Jenny and thereby acknowledging his feelings permits an easier way of introducing diversion, without ignoring or dehumanising Bobby's feelings and emotions.

Drug treatments for Alzheimer's disease

Although there is no known cure for Alzheimer's disease, there are drugs available which may slow down the effects of the dementia upon the person by diminishing the symptoms for a period of time. The drugs maintain the person's level of functioning by helping cognitive symptoms such as memory loss and may also have a beneficial effect on behaviour (including mood). However, the underlying disease process is still progressing.

These drugs are called acetylcholinesterase inhibitors and are effective in the mild to moderate stages. During the process of Alzheimer's disease there is a depletion of a chemical in the brain called acetylcholine which helps nerve cells to communicate with each other. This chemical is normally broken down by an enzyme called acetylcholinesterase. The drugs work by inhibiting (or blocking) this enzyme and thus increasing the amount of acetlycholine in the brain.

There are currently three drugs licensed in the UK for the symptomatic treatment of Alzheimer's disease: donepezil, galantamine and rivastigmine. Memantine is currently licensed for the treatment of moderate to severe Alzheimer's disease. Memantine blocks a neurotransmitter (glutamate), which is released in excessive amounts when brain cells are damaged by Alzheimer's disease. Although this drug is licensed in the UK it is not recommended as a treatment option for people with Alzheimer's disease except as part of clinical trials (NICE, 2006).

Not all people with dementia will respond to treatment. Only a third will show improvement, a third will not deteriorate and a third will have no response and continue to deteriorate. You might come across an individual on a drug treatment for their dementia in the hospital or community setting. It is useful to be aware of the potential side effects of this commonly used medication. These include:

- Appetite disturbance
- Diarrhoea
- Drowsiness
- Stomach cramps
- Nausea
- Nightmares
- Increased confusion
- Urinary incontinence

Treatment for vascular dementia

There are currently no drugs available for the treatment of vascular dementia. However, if the clinical picture suggests a mixed form of dementia then acetylcholinesterase inhibitors may be considered. The main aim of treatment for vascular dementia is to reduce the risk of further strokes through the modification of cardiovascular risk factors (see *Table 3*). However, it is important to remember that these factors should be addressed in all people with dementia regardless of its form. Practitioners are in an ideal position to advise individuals on stroke reduction strategies as they constitute the foundation stones of healthy living policy.

Challenging behaviour in dementia

Challenging behaviour takes several forms in dementia as detailed in *Table 4*. Although changes in the brain as a result of dementia may cause behavioural problems, in reality there are several reasons why patients might exhibit such behaviour. It may be more helpful to regard the patient's actions as a form of communication.

Factors from a person's background such as personality, occupational and leisure activities and a person's habitual way of responding to stress may be fundamental to their current behaviour. These include medical and physiological factors such as pain, hunger, thirst, need for the toilet, need for exercise, side effects to medication and increased confusion. One or a combination of the above factors may cause problem behaviour or exacerbate existing behavioural patterns.

Is the behaviour triggered by emotion such as boredom, anger, anxiety or insecurity? Hospitalisation and care home placement are distressing enough for people without dementia but such a change can be catastrophic and disorientating for people with the condition.

Changes within the brain may cause functional deficits such as an inability to carry out complex tasks, which leads to frustration.

Changes within the brain can affect perception and spatial awareness. This may result in a patient getting into the wrong bed or being unable to put their clothes on in the right order.

Environmental factors can contribute towards challenging behaviour and include ward layout, proximity to other people, lacking control over routine (such as bedtime and meal times), being in a strange place, unfamiliar tasks (such as blood pressure measurement) and sensory stimulation overload which might include the general business of a ward environment and unknown faces and smells. Transition from home to a care home can be particularly confusing for people with dementia who may be described disparagingly as 'wanderers' during the first few weeks. However it is natural for somebody who is in a new place (and has forgotten they have been told they are moving home) to want to return 'home'.

What can be done to minimise and manage challenging behaviour?
Dementia can affect expressive and receptive language. As the disease progresses communication becomes less verbal and people use more body language. Communication is made up of 3 components: 55% body language; 38% tone and pitch of voice; 7% words we use. Try doing the following to improve communication between yourself and a person with dementia:

- Try to catch and hold attention of your patient before starting to communicate
- Allow time for unhurried interaction
- Keep environmental noise to a minimum, e.g. turn TV down
- Avoid negative body language. People with dementia will pick up on hostile body language. If you raise your voice they may respond in a similar fashion. Likewise, if you are kind and gentle, they are likely to follow suit
- Remain pleasant, calm, confident and supportive

Table 3. Modification of vascular risk factors

Treatment of strokes and transient ischaemic attacks (TIA's)
Blood pressure control People with dementia and carers should be encouraged to take anti-hypertensive medication and have their blood pressure checked regularly
Management and treatment of high blood cholesterol (hypercholesterolaemia). This may be achieved through following a low fat diet alone or in combination with the prescription of a statin
Modification of alcohol intake People with dementia should be advised to drink in moderation, i.e. no more than two units of alcohol per day. Alcohol can exacerbate memory problems when taken in excess
Smoking cessation People with dementia should be encouraged to give up smoking. Appropriate guidance regarding smoking cessation clinics and methods to give up smoking should be given
Physical exercise People with dementia should be advised to exercise regularly such as 30 minutes per day. This does not have to be intensive gym activity but could simply mean a walk in a local park
Diet People with dementia should be advised to eat a varied low salt, low fat diet. Referral to a dietician may be helpful

Table 4. Examples of challenging behaviour in dementia

Behaviour	Example
Difficult behaviour	Patient refuses to cooperate with therapy
Aggressive/disruptive behaviour	Verbal or physical aggression to others, destroying objects around others or self (e.g. trying to pull out catheters,) wandering, rummaging though lockers, interfering with other patients
Deficient behaviour	Patient may be hypoactive, apathetic or withdrawn

- Maintain eye contact with your patient
- Use short sentences
- Speak slowly and wait for response
- Ask only one question at a time
- Keep the pitch of your voice low but ensure patient can hear you
- Point, touch, show, initiate a movement for the patient

- Avoid challenging patient or do so in an non-threatening way
- Double check instructions to ensure understanding
- Answer repetitive questions consistently
- Use written instructions
- Ensure patient has access to sensory aids such as hearing aid and glasses. Sensory deprivation affects communication and may exacerbate confusion
- Avoid confrontation. Withdraw for a few minutes rather than persevere causing possible aggression to mount

Coping strategies in challenging behaviour

- Identify underlying cause of any acute confusion (delirium) through full history (from carer/GP), medical examinations and investigations, e.g. urinalysis, blood tests
- Encourage regular visits from carer/relatives as they are often a reassuring presence
- Try and ensure continuity of care through same care team and named nurse. Establishing a rapport with your patient enables them to get to know you and thus will give them security and trust
- Find out a little about your patient. What did they do for a living? What is their normal routine? Does the carer have any usual coping strategies to share with you?
- Carers and relatives know your patients best and can often explain unusual behaviour and how to manage it. Long-term memory is preserved until much later in dementia so talking to your patient about the past is a stimulating pastime. It also shows your patient you value them
- Avoid neuroleptics and sedating drugs (such as haloperidol) if possible as they may exacerbate confusion and increase risk of falls. Medication is a last resort
- Ensure side rail policy is adhered to. Bed rails are not appropriate for every patient, e.g. patients with dementia who try to get out of bed may climb over side rails. They may need to be nursed on a mattress on the floor. All healthcare organisations should have a side rail policy
- Document triggers to behaviour and record type, frequency and severity of behaviour
- Situations tend to escalate so recognising triggers to challenging behaviour might prevent a full-scale incident. For example: a patient might become aggressive during personal care provided by a male nurse, therefore ensure a female nurse cares for patient
- Try and ensure any tubing/venflons are well secured and hidden from sight
- Patients with dementia may not understand the need for a urinary catheter and may try and pull it out. Ensure underwear is worn and

tubing is securely attached. Leg bags might be better tolerated
- Ensure lighting is appropriate. People with dementia might get confused about shadows and the dark. They may find it distressing so sleeping with dim lights on might be preferred
- Attend to bowel and bladder elimination. Observe for signs of dehydration and constipation as both are implicated in delirium
- Ensure your patient has adequate dietary and fluid intake. Ensure food and drinks are within reach of patient and assess their ability to eat and drink independently. Make food manageable and assist with feeding/ drinking as appropriate
- Place patient close to nurses station (if in hospital)
- Try and provide stimulating activities for your patient. Consider referral to the activities co-ordinator.

Delirium

Delirium is a common problem seen in all settings. It is a condition that comes on very rapidly, affecting a person's brain for a very short period of time and can cause confusion, restless behaviour, drowsiness and sometimes a complete change in personality. It is often referred to as acute confusional state. It can occur at any age but is more common with increasing age and with the presence of dementia. It may be distressing for individuals, relatives and staff members. Unfortunately it often goes unrecognised by uninformed health providers. There is usually an underlying medical cause of delirium and thus it should be regarded as a medical emergency.

Features of delirium

If the person you care for shows features similar to the symptoms described below report them to your senior colleagues. You might have picked up on the first signs of a potentially life-threatening illness:

- Sudden worsening of mental state and behaviour over a period of hours or days that fluctuates
- Hyperactivity and agitation. Person with delirium might shout out or become aggressive
- Hypoactivity (withdrawal, lack of motivation, drowsiness, difficulty rousing person with delirium)
- Unusual behaviour such as hallucinations (seeing or hearing things), wandering, mistaking other objects for the toilet such as a waste paper basket.

- Symptoms worse towards evening/night
- Disorientation, i.e. not knowing where you are, who you are or what time period you are in
- Disturbed level of consciousness, i.e. increased drowsiness or restlessness. Often fluctuations between the two
- Difficulty focusing/concentrating or understanding what is being said
- Memory problems-commonly short-term memory is affected so person with delirium may not realise they are in hospital

Table 5 shows some of the risk factors for delirium. By being aware of high risk patients and looking out for signs of delirium you might be able to reduce the severity and duration of the episode of delirium and might even prevent its occurrence in some individuals.

Common causes of delirium

- Infection
- Neurological, such as stroke, epilepsy, acute brain injury
- Cardiological, such as heart attack
- Respiratory, such as pulmonary embolism, hypoxia
- Endocrine/metabolic, such as hypothyroidism, hypoglycaemia and hyperglycaemia
- Drugs (legal and illegal substances), such as tramadol and morphine
- Alcohol withdrawal

Up to 60% care home residents develop delirium at some point. Up to 24% of older patients admitted to hospital have delirium and up to 56% will develop delirium during their hospital stay. Up to 42% of patients who have fractured their hip develop delirium by day 3 post-operatively. Diagnosis of delirium is missed in up to 70% cases. Up to a third of cases may be preventable.

Table 5.   Risk factors for delirium

Advanced age
Severe illness (e.g. in critical care)
Dementia
Physical frailty
Admission with dehydration/infection
Visual impairment
Surgery
Certain drug treatments such as anticholinergics (such as oxybutynin) and opiates (such as morphine)
Alcohol excess

Case study 1: community

Mrs S is a 92 year-old lady with dementia. She has been a resident at a care home for the past 5 years and is well known to the staff. Mrs S is usually friendly, outgoing and co-operative with her care. She is usually continent and can use the toilet independently. She also loves her food.

Over the past two days her named carer (Mary) has noticed a distinct change in Mrs B. She has been reluctant to get out of bed and has become snappy and irritable. She has gone off her food and tells the care staff to leave her alone. She has also become incontinent of urine. Mary told the nurse in charge that she was worried about the sudden change in Mrs S's behaviour. The nurse took her temperature and it was raised. She also tested her urine and it contained protein, blood and nitrates.

The GP was called and he prescribed Mrs S a course of antibiotics for a urinary tract infection. Staff encouraged Mrs S to take plenty of fluid to prevent dehydration and ensured she did not become constipated. Within a week she had returned back to her old self and her appetite was better and her incontinence was resolved.

Diagnosis: Hypoactive delirium as a result of urinary tract infection

Case study 2: hospital

Mr B is a 77 year-old gentleman who lives alone and is usually fully independent. He wears glasses and is quite deaf but does not have a history of dementia or memory impairment. He recently fell whilst getting off the bus and sustained a fractured hip. He was admitted to hospital and underwent a hip replacement. When Mr B returned from the recovery ward he was disorientated, agitated and kept trying to pull his drip out. He was very confused. He shouted out at night for his wife (who had passed away). Over the next few days, as Mr B started to recover from the operation, the confusion slowly resolved. On discharge Mr B told the ward staff he remembered feeling confused and angry and was acutely embarrassed about it. He was also concerned that this might happen again. The staff explained to him that the anaesthetic and surgery had made him behave in this way and his sensory impairment (visual and hearing) increased his risk of developing delirium. The ward doctor ensured Mr B had a follow-up appointment not only to check his physical recovery but also to ensure he was psychologically recovering from this traumatic episode.

Diagnosis: Hyperactive delirium as a result of anaesthesia and surgery

Case study 3: intermediate care unit

Mrs J is an 82 year-old lady who suffers from mild Alzheimer's disease. She was recently transferred to the local intermediate care unit following a successful operation to remove a cancerous tumour from her bowel. She was prescribed tramadol for severe osteoarthritis pain of her knees. However, three days after her admission the night nurses reported that Mrs J had become uncharacteristically disruptive. She was calling out at night and appeared to be hallucinating. By day, Mrs J had become withdrawn and reluctant to engage with physiotherapy. She was unable to hold a full conversation with staff and her attention appeared to be drifting. After a medical review it was felt that Mrs J was delirious due to a combination of the tramadol and also constipation as a consequence of the drug. The tramadol was stopped, paracetamol was given for the knee pain with good effect and the constipation was treated with laxatives. Over the next few days she recovered. .

Diagnosis: Mixed delirium as a result of adverse drug side effects and constipation

Depression

Depression is a common illness that can have a significant negative impact on the quality of life of older people. More than two million people over the age of 65 have symptoms of depression and of those with clinical depression only 15% get treated (Age Concern, 2008). Current guidance by NICE (2007) advises on the treatment and management of depression and related conditions. It advocates screening in primary care and general hospitals for depression in high risk groups such as those with a previous history of depression, significant physical illnesses causing disability or other mental health problems including dementia. This guidance provides advice regarding pharmacological management of depression and non-pharmacological management of the condition including cognitive behavioural therapy (NICE, 2007).

What is depression?

Depression is a mood disorder, which is often expressed as sadness, despair or discouragement. Depression can occur in dementia and the symptoms of depression can also be mistaken for those of dementia. Older people with depression often present with physical complaints such as constipation when they are suffering from a mental health problem.

Signs and symptoms of depression include:

- Mental deterioration such as forgetfulness, difficulty thinking and making decisions
- Emotional deterioration such as tearfulness, negative thoughts, excessive or unnecessary worry, low self esteem, guilt, hopelessness, thoughts of death or suicide
- Loss of motivation, withdrawal, self neglect
- Disturbed sleep pattern. Patients with depression often find it difficult getting off to sleep and wake early
- Fatigue
- Movement disorder such as slowness, retardation, agitation
- Weight loss, reduced appetite and other physical symptoms such as constipation and gastrointestinal problems
- Loss of libido

The symptoms of depression, delirium and dementia can overlap and can also co-exist but it is important to distinguish between the conditions as depression and delirium are potentially treatable disorders (*Table 6*).

Causes of depression

The causes of depression are not completely understood but may well be a combination of genetic and environmental factors.

Genetics

Some types of depression run in families suggesting that some elements of depression are inherited. There may be some evidence to suggest there are differences in brain structure in people who are depressed (Blows, 2003). In people experiencing depression there are changes in their messaging chemicals or neurotransmitters. These chemicals are:

- Serotonin — has a role in maintaining normal patterns of appetite, sleep and sexual activity
- Noradrenaline — helps to regulate mood and energy
- Dopamine — is thought to have a role in the acquisition of pleasure

Drugs that rebalance these chemicals can help relieve symptoms.

Depressive disorders are more common in patients with physical illness (McHale, 2003). Some medical problems have a stronger association with

Table 6.   Distinguishing features between depression, dementia and delirium

	Depression	**Dementia**	**Delirium**
History	Onset and decline often rapid with identifiable triggers or life event, for example a bereavement	Vague insidious onset, symptoms progress slowly	Sudden onset over hours and days with fluctuations
Symptoms	Obvious at an early stage	Might go unnoticed for years	Obvious if hyperactive delirium but may be harder to recognise if 'hypoactive' delirium (e.g. apathy)
	Subjective complaints of memory loss	Lack of insight. Attempts to hide problems or is unaware. Often disorientated to time, place and person. Processing of external and internal information impaired	Disorientation to time, place and person. Short-term memory impaired. Processing of external and internal information impaired
	Symptoms often worse in the morning	Confusion worse in the evening (sundowning)	Confusion worse at night
Consciousness	Normal	Normal	Clouding consciousness (impaired attention)
Mental state	Distressed/unhappy	Possible labile mood	Emotional lability anxiety, fear, depression, aggression
	Variability in cognitive performance	Consistent cognitive performance (though not as consistent in people with Lewy Body dementia)	Variability in cognitive performance
Delusions/ hallucinations	Rare	Delusions common. Hallucinations rare in early stage dementia	Common
Psychomotor disturbance	May get psychomotor retardation if depression is severe	Psychomotor disturbance evident in later stages	Psychomotor disturbance-purposeless apathetic or hyperactive

psychiatric illnesses. This is important for practitioners to consider when identifying patients who may be at higher risk of developing depression. Certain physical illnesses that are particularly linked to depression include: Parkinson's disease; dementia; multiple sclerosis; heart disease; stroke; high blood pressure; and hypothyroidism.

The side effects of some prescribed drugs also may also induce depression. Two classes of drugs in particular may be implicated (Patten and Barbui, 2004: beta-blockers (commonly used to treat heart problems and hypertension) such as atenolol, propanolol and corticosteroids such as dexamathasone and hydrocortisone. Practitioners are advised to tell patients to obtain further advice from a doctor if they develop depressive symptoms after starting new medication.

Taking part in fewer activities or having fewer interests can cause depression, or may happen because of depression. Social isolation as a result of caring or physical ill health are examples.

A stressful or upsetting life event can cause a persistent low mood, low self-esteem and feelings of hopelessness about the future. Examples include bereavement, divorce and redundancy.

Screening for depression

All practitioners have a role to play in identifying patients who may be depressed. There are several easy to use assessment tools to assist with the assessment process. A commonly used tool is the Beck Depression Inventory (Beck, 1961) which is a self-administered questionnaire. The Geriatric Depression Scale is also a quick and effective way of detecting symptoms of depression (Yesavage et al, 1982).

Treatment

Treatment usually involves a combination of drugs, talking therapies and self-help.

Mild depression
Often mild depression will not need any specific treatment. Physical activity, structured routines, healthy diet and a good amount of sleep may alleviate mild symptoms (Healy, 2005).

Moderate depression
If mild depression is not improving or a patient has moderate depression medical advice should be sought and patients may be prescribed antidepressant therapy or a talking treatment such as cognitive behavioural therapy or counselling.

Severe depression

Patients with severe depression may receive antidepressant therapy in addition to a talking treatment. In extremely severe cases where depression persists (or the situation is life threatening) electro-convulsive therapy may be considered.

Antidepressant therapy

Commonly used anti-depressants are those called selected serotonin reuptake inhibitors (SSRIs). As mentioned earlier one possible cause of depression may be linked to a reduction in the chemical serotonin. SSRIs work by increasing the natural levels of serotonin in the brain and thereby lift mood. Examples of SSRIs include fluoxetine, paroxetine and citalopram. Potential side effects are nausea, sleep disturbance and increased anxiety.

Other forms of antidepressants include tricyclic antidepressants (TCAs) such as amitriptyline, and serotonin-norepinephrine reuptake inhibitors (SSNIs) such as venlafaxine.

It is very important that patients are given comprehensive information about their medication, covering possible side effects and also informing patients that antidepressants can take up to four weeks to take effect. Efficacy of treatment should be monitored regularly and patients should be advised that cessation of treatment should only be done with medical advice.

Caring for the carers

There are approximately six million carers in England and Wales (Office for National Statistics, 2003). Carers provide the vast majority of health and community care. Nearly two thirds of carers look after someone with a disability: 7% care for someone with a mental disability and 15% care for someone with a physical and a mental disability.

Practitioners are in an ideal position to signpost carers to the most appropriate support services.

- The Alzheimer's Society provides advice on all aspects of dementia care and all forms of dementia. www.alzheimers.org.uk or telephone 0845 300 0336
- Rethink is a mental health charity which offers support to people affected by mental ill health and their carers through provision of literature, support groups and an informative website. www.rethink.org or telephone 0845 456 0455
- Carers UK is a nationwide organisation providing information for carers ranging from carers rights and welfare benefits to where to access respite care www.carersuk.org or telephone 0207 490 8818

Conclusion

This chapter has shown practitioners how common mental health disorders are in older people. As an ageing population, the prevalence of such conditions is expected to rise significantly, practitioners should feel confident in recognising the signs and symptoms of three common mental health problems in older people, namely dementia, delirium and depression, in addition to having a sound understanding of the management of each condition. The needs of carers have been highlighted and practitioners should be able to signpost carers to the appropriate organisation for ongoing support. It is hoped that practitioners in all settings will feel able to apply the knowledge acquired here to their individual workplace.

Age Concern (2008) *Undiagnosed, Untreated, At Risk. The Experience of Older People with Depression.* Age Concern, London

Alzheimer's Society (2008) Information Sheet 456: *The Brain and Behaviour.* Alzheimer's Society, London

Bagley H Cordingley L, Burns A, Godlove Mozley C, Sutcliffe C, Challis, D, Huxley P (2000) Recognition of depression by staff in nursing and residential homes. *Journal of Clinical Nursing* **9 (3)** 445-450

Blows W (2003) *The Biological Basis of Nursing: Mental Health.* Routledge, London

Clare L, Woods RT (2004) Cognitive training and cognitive rehabilitation for people with early stage Alzheimer's disease: a review. *Neuropsychological Rehabilitation* **14**:385–401

Cox S, Cook A (2002) Caring for people with dementia at the end. In: Hockley, J, Clark D, eds. *Palliative Care for Older People in Care Homes.* Open University Press, Buckingham: 86-103

Department of Health and the Care Services Improvement Partnership (2005) *Everybody's Business — Integrated Mental Health Services for Older Adults: a Service Development Guide.* DH, London

DH (2008) *End of Life Care Strategy — Promoting High Quality Care for all Adults at the End of Life.* DH, London

DH (2009) *Living well with Dementia: A National Dementia Strategy.* DH, London

Hobson P (2007) Understanding Dementia: Neurological Impairment. *British Journal of Healthcare Assistants* **1(7):** 294–6

Inouye S, Bogardus S, Charpentier P, Leo-Summers L, Acampora D, Holford T, Cooney LA (1999) Multicomponent Intervention to Prevent Delirium in Hospitalized Older Patients *New England Journal of Medicine* **340**(9): 669-676

Janicki M, Dalton AJ (2002) Prevalence of Dementia and Impact on Intellectual Disability

Services. *Mental Retardation* **38**: 276-288.

Kitwood T (1997) *Dementia Reconsidered: The Person Comes First*. Open University Press, Buckingham

Knapp M, Prince M, Albanese E, Banerjee S, Dhanasiri S, Fernandez JL, Ferri C, McCrone P (2007) *Dementia UK: A report into the prevalence and cost of dementia*. London School of Economics and the Institute of Psychiatry, London

Lehr RP (2006) The Brain Map *http://www.neuroskills.com/brain.shtml*. Accessed May 5th 2009

MacHale ,S (2002) Managing depression in physical illness. *Advances in Psychiatric Treatment* **8**: 297-305

National Council for Palliative Care (2009) *Out of the Shadows. End of life care for people with dementia*. The National Council for Palliative Care, London.

National Institute for Health and Clinical Excellence (2006) *NICE Guideline 42: Quick Reference Guide: Dementia. Supporting People with Dementia and their Carers in Health and Social Care*. NICE, London

National Institute for Clinical Excellence (2007) *Depression*. NICE, London

Patten SB, Barbui C (2004) Drug-induced depression. A systematic review to inform clinical practice. *Psychotherapy and Psychosomatics* **73**:207-215

Royal College of Psychiatrists (2005) *Who cares wins: improving the outcome for older people admitted to the general hospital: guidelines for the development of liaison mental health services for older people*. Royal College of Psychiatrists, London

Royal College of Psychiatrists (2006) *Guidelines for the Prevention, Management and Diagnosis of Delirium in Older People in Hospital*. Royal College of Psychiatrists. London people admitted to t

Royal College of Psychiatrists (2008) *A collective responsibility to act now on ageing and mental health: a consensus statement http://www.its-services.org.uk/silo/files/consensus-statement.pdf*. Accessed 12th May 2009

Singleton N, Maung NA, Cowie J *et al* (2002) *Mental Health of Carers*. Office for National Statistics, London

UK Inquiry into Mental Health and Well-being in Later Life (2007) *Improving Services and Support for Older People with Mental Health Problems: The final report from the UK inquiry* Age Concern England

Walsh D (2006*) Dementia Care Training Manual for Staff working in Nursing and Residential Settings*. Jessica Kingsley Publishers, London

Yesavage JA, Brink TL, Rose TL, *et al.* (1982) Development and validation of a geriatric depression screening scale: a preliminary report. *Journal of Psychiatric Research* **17**: 37-49

CHAPTER 13

Caring for the person who has a learning disability

Chris Barber

There are between 1.2 and 1.4 million people in the UK who have a diagnosis of learning disability (Peate and Fearne, 2006; Clark and Griffiths, 2008). This figure of 1.4 million breaks down to 800,000 adults age over 20 (Peate and Fearns, 2006) and 600,000 children and young adults under the age of 20. This equates to nearly 1 and a half times the total population of Birmingham and about 20% of the total population of London. On top of that, the number of adults with a learning disability is set to rise by 14% to 900,000 by 2021 (Peate and Fearne, 2006).

Put very simply, a person with a learning disability is another way of saying a person with an intellectual deficit. The legal definition according to the Mental Health Act 1983 (DH, 1983) is that learning disability is an arrested or incomplete development of mind. A more helpful definition of learning disabilities can be found in Peate and Fearne (2006). It is worth repeating it here. A person has a learning disability if the following are present:

- A significantly reduced ability to understand new or complex information or to learn new skills
- A reduced ability to cope independently
- Disability started before adulthood with a lasting effect on development.

Many conditions such as schizophrenia and other forms of psychosis and Alzheimer's disease and other forms of dementia could be argued to meet the first two criteria but not the last point, and so does not qualify as forms of learning disability unless the psychosis started in childhood. However, Clark and Griffiths (2008) include such conditions as acquired brain injury, dementia and some forms of severe mental health issues such as schizophrenia as forms of 'learning disability'. An acquired brain injury is an injury affecting the brain caused through physical trauma such as being hit by a moving car or through eating or drinking something that is toxic to the brain and other parts of the central nervous system. Yet, some forms of pervasive developmental disorders such as autism and Asperger's syndrome are generally seen as learning disabilities and people with these have services provided by learning disability teams, which includes psychologists and psychiatrists specialising in learning disabilities.

It could be argued that the meaning of learning disability is intimately connected to and results in labels such as mental defective, mental sub-normality, mental handicap, idiots, and imbeciles. The use of language forms the definition of learning disability, and also informs the on-going debates on the meaning of care-giving and care for those who have a learning disability. Over time these debates facilitate changes in the understanding of learning disability by helping others to think about what it is like to have and to live with a learning disability. This in turn influences the type of services made available to the learning disabled and also helps us to focus on the overall of services required.

Development of understanding

The history, meaning and understanding of, and care for, those with a learning disability have changed radically over the centuries, with its history being intimately bound to and shaped by the use of language. An example of this is the change in the registered nurse qualification. Although the current registration is Registered Nurse (Learning Disability), when I qualified at the end of 1989 my qualification was Registered Nurse (Mental Handicap), and my lecturers' qualification (one of whom qualified only 10 years before me) was Registered Nurse (Mental subnormality).

So what is the history of learning disability? I am indebted here to Farmer et al (1993) for these historical notes.

Eighteenth century
Before the end of the end of the eighteenth century very little was known about learning disability as a mental or health condition. It is probably safe to assume that those people with a learning disability who survived beyond birth and childhood would have been cared for, probably somewhat brutally, either at home or in religious institutions. Many would have become tramps or 'knights of the road'. They would have been seen as simpletons, village idiots or even, in some cases, holy and saintly innocents who would have been seen as being very close to God through their simplicity and innocence and treated accordingly.

Nineteenth century
Scientific interest in the diagnosis and care of people with a mental problem grew at the end of the eighteenth and early nineteenth centuries as psychological medicine advanced alongside an increasing interest in eugenics

(the science of the improvement of the human race through genetics) mental 'defectives' were seen as extremely fertile and a threat to racial quality. In the nineteenth century compulsory basic education was also established. This enabled those with a learning disability to be seen as separate from those with a sensory impairment resulting in the need for children with a learning disability to be educated in special classes, a practice which is evident even today. Care for those with a learning disability were seen as being best met in institutions/asylums and most, if not all, were located in rural settings.

Twentieth century

The twentieth century was marked by a large number of Royal Commissions, Government reports and Acts of Parliament. Examples of these include the 1908 Royal Commission and the 1913 Mental Deficiency Act which allowed for and even imposed segregation of the 'mentally defective' and mentally ill into self-contained institutions as an alternative to enforced sterilisation. Although isolated experiments in 'community care existed in the late nineteenth century, it was not until the 1957 Royal Commission and the 1959 Mental Health Act that the emphasis of care for those with a learning disability seriously moved from institutional to community care and more flexible care provision. Improvements in care served as the focus for the 1971 and the 1979 Government reports, improvements based on 'normalisation theories'. The 1983 Mental Health Act provided a legal definition of mental impairment.

Twenty first century

The twenty first century started with the publication of the first White Paper on learning disabilities for two decades, *Valuing People*, with its emphasis on inclusion, participation, rights, respect and dignity (DH 2001). We have thus progressed over the last 250 years, albeit somewhat slowly and hesitantly, from fear and isolation, through tolerance and then acceptance, to an integration where those with a learning disability are seen largely as valued citizens with equal rights to everybody else. It will be interesting to see how we develop from here in the coming decades.

Health conditions and learning disabilities

Clark and Griffiths (2008) suggest that physical and mental health needs and problems prevalent in people with a learning disability often go unrecognised. This could be for any number of reasons including a lack of resources to meet these needs, a lack of awareness and understanding that those with a learning disability do actually have the same health needs and problems as everyone else within society, and an identified lack of training received by care professionals such as nurses and doctors. Indeed, one adult trained nurse betrayed this lack of knowledge and understanding when she once asked me: '*Well, what is this disease called Asperger's?*' This lack of professional knowledge and understanding indicates that those with a learning disability are not having their needs met by the caring profession.

The following is a brief description of some of the health conditions that people who have a learning disability might additionally have (Higgins and O'Toole, 2008).

- **Neurological disorders**: These include epilepsy, some forms of behavioural disorders and mental health problems such as schizophrenia arising from brain damage
- **Sensory impairment**: There is a very strong association between both visual and hearing impairment and those with a learning disability. Between 20-30% of adults with learning disabilities have a visual impairment and around 40% have a hearing impairment
- **Cardiovascular disease**: Cardiovascular disease is regularly reported. Van den Akker et al (2006) found that 14% of people with a learning disability were diagnosed with cardiac disease, and between 14% and 20% had coronary artery disease. These made coronary heart disease the second highest cause of death for people with a learning disability.
- **Endocrine system**: Thyroid problems and diabetes are noted by Higgins and O'Toole (2008) to be high in people with learning disabilities. Thyroid problems are a common issue in Down's syndrome for example.
- **Reproductive system**: Amongst the fairly common reproductive issues with people with a learning disability include hypogonadism in both men and women. Undescended testes in men with Down's syndrome, for example, appears to be quite common.
- **Urinary system**: People with learning disabilities seem to be prone to urinary tract infection. Possible reasons include perceived poor personal hygiene and problems associated with incontinence, and insufficient fluid intake.
- **Muscular/skeletal system**: problems with bones and muscles are quite common in those with cerebral palsy and forms of muscle degenerative disorders. These could include spinal deformities such as kyphosis (outward curvature), scoliosis (left or right curvature) and lordosis (lumbar or cervical inward curvature)
- **Oral health care**: Due to a number of factors including poor or non-existent oral care and hygiene and poor cleaning technique, those

with learning disabilities tend to have a greater number of oral health problems than the general population (Shapira et al, 1998)

- **Nutrition and feeding problems**: There are a number of eating and drinking problems that can be associated with multiple learning and physical disabilities including problems with chewing and swallowing, pica (the eating on non-nutritious substances such as dirt, stones, clothing, etc.), constipation and other bowel disorders and behavioural problems
- **Sexual health**: People with a learning disability are at greater risk of sexual abuse and coercion into prostitution than the general population, with associated increased risks of pregnancy and sexually transmitted infections
- **Mental health**: There is a general agreement now that those with a learning disability experience the same forms of mental health problems such as depression, bipolar mood disorders and schizophrenia, to not only the same extent as but probably more commonly than the general population.

Lifestyle and learning disability

There are a number of other major issues that could negatively affect the lives and wellbeing of those with a learning disability. These may include, amongst many others, the issues in *Box 1*:

Box 1 Issues affecting people who have a learning disability

- Education
- Communication
- Social engagement
- Human rights
- Challenging behaviour
- Attitudes towards those with a learning disability
- Provision of services
- Parenting and learning disabilities
- Advocacy
- Legislation
- Health action plans
- Person centred approach
- Power
- Sexuality
- Inclusion and exclusion
- Spirituality

Some of these may seem fairly mundane and even trivial, whilst others such as education, employment and communication may seem hugely important. However important, trivial or in-between though many of these issues are, they will all impact upon the lives and wellbeing of those with a learning disability and their carers, carers that includes the parents, siblings and the extended family of those with a learning disability. The next section highlights some of the roles that the healthcare assistant may well be asked to undertake in order to improve the lives and wellbeing of those who have a learning disability, and also that of their families.

The health and social care assistant has a number of roles in ensuring a high quality of care is given to people with learning disabilities. I am not going to suggest ways that you could meet the specific needs of specific service users in specific settings as there are far too many individuals with individual needs in individual environments for that to be feasible or appropriate here. The following role suggestions are deliberately general but hopefully not vague and may prove to be a helpful underpinning of more specific input with specific service users.

The first, and possibly the most important of these for you as the healthcare assistant giving direct care is to be aware of and be familiar and comfortable with the main features of and issues facing those with a learning disability. This could be a mammoth task: where do you start? Well, there are a number of journals available that range from the more general-purpose nursing and social care journals through to the more specialised journals, some more helpful and useful than others. Amongst the former you will find *Social Work Today, Nursing Standard, British Journal of Nursing, British Journal of Health Care Assistants and Nursing Times* and amongst the latter you will find the *Journal of Intellectual Disability Research* and *Learning Disability Practice*. There are also a large number of books available.

There are a number of voluntary sector organisations in the field of learning disabilities such as Mencap, the National Autistic Society and the Rathbone Society, which will be only too pleased to provide a wide range of basic and accessible information. The Royal College of Nursing Learning Disability Forum will also provide information on learning disability.

There are also a number of courses which you could attend. These range from the NVQ-based Learning Disability Awards Framework (LDAF) through to more academic short and long duration courses. Universities that run learning disability nurse training will have details of such courses.

It is important to learn how to communicate with people with a learning disability. Many would find verbal communication difficult if not impossible either due to their learning disability or because of an accompanying physical disability which may prevent the person from verbally communicating. As an illustration of this, just think of the possible physical problems that a person who has had a stroke may experience due to articulating sounds through tongue control for example. To help you communicate better with people with a learning disability you could attend a short course on Makaton. Makaton is a sign language used by those with a learning disability and which is very similar to the British Sign Language used by those who have a hearing impairment.

Finally, at all times you must treat the person with a learning disability with the same respect, courtesy and dignity that you would expect for yourself or that you would show to other non-learning disabled service users, regardless of the level or severity of their disability, communication ability and the environment or setting where you work. To do anything other than that as a basic minimum is unprofessional, unethical and can never be justified. People with a learning disability are human beings first and foremost and, as such, demand and deserve the right to be treated accordingly. They are not perpetual children trapped in an adult body. If the person before you is an adult who has a learning disability then approach them respectfully and as an adult. You may and possibly will have to modify how you approach and communicate with people with a learning disability but that must not be at the price of denying them their humanity and uniqueness. Likewise, do not fall into the trap of approaching and treating all those with a learning disability in the same way. Each person with a learning disability is as individual and unique as you and I, with their own individual sets of health and social care needs, hopes, desires, expectations and history. Approach, communicate with and treat them accordingly.

Conclusion

I hope that the aim of this chapter of in stimulating a foundation understanding of learning disability issues has been achieved. If you leave this short chapter with one thing to remember it is this: it is not what a person looks like, or a diagnostic label that might be attached to them, that matters. It is who the person is. Someone who has a learning disability is, first and foremost, a human being and has the right to be treated accordingly.

Clark L, Griffiths P (2008) *Learning disability and other intellectual impairments*. John Wiley, Chichester

Department of Health (1983) *The Mental Health Act*. The Stationary Office, London

Department of Health (2001) *Valuing people: A new strategy for learning disability for the 21st Century*. DH, London

Farmer R, Rohde J, Sacks B (1993) *Changing services for people with learning disabilities.*

Chapman and Hall, London

Higgins S, O'Toole (2008) Meeting the health of people with intellectual impairment. In: Clark L, Griffiths P eds. *Learning disability and other intellectual impairments*. John Wiley, Chichester

Mencap (2007) *Death by indifference*. Mencap, London

Peate I, Fearns D (2006) *Caring for people with learning disabilities*. John Wiley, Chichester

Shapira J, Efrat J, Berkey D, Mann J (1998) Dental health profile of a population with mental retardation in Israel. *Specialist Care in Dentistry* **18:** 149–55

Van den Akker M, Maaskant M van den Meijden R (2006) Cardiac diseases in people with intellectual disability. *Journal of intellectual disability* **50**(7): 515–22

CHAPTER 14

Spirituality

Chris Barber

Spirituality has become a highly salient term, not only in relation to nursing, health and social care, but within society in general (McSherry, 2007).

The meaning of the word 'spirituality' is like one of those 'how long is a piece of string' conundrums. There are many possibilities, so many questions and answers depending on personal, ethical, religious and philosophical perspectives.

Spirituality is not the same as religion, although it may be linked to religion. It encompasses a standing still in order to reflect on what is to be fully human, whilst also a journey of change, a journey which has no end.

The word 'spirituality' is based on the Latin *spirare*, to breathe, the act of breathing being vital to the existence and continuation of life. Spirituality should not be considered to be purely based on egocentric (self-centred) thoughts. The Greek word for 'spiritual' is *koinonia* which means living so as to meet the needs of another, a passion for the good or welfare of another.

McSherry (2007) gives a number of definitions of spirituality which include:

- Spirituality is my being, my inner person. It is who I am. It is me expressed through my body, my thinking, my judgements and my creativity
- Spirituality is a quality that goes beyond religious affiliation, that strives for inspirations, reverence, awe, meaning and purpose
- Spirituality is a way of understanding existence
- Spirituality is a search for the meaning of life.

There are many varied and diverse attempts to define spirituality. We all have our own understanding of what spirituality is and we all experience and live this understanding in different and personal ways. However, it could be suggested that there is sufficient meaning in common to come up with an over-arching definition of spirituality.

Difference between spirituality and religion

Whilst every one has a spiritual dimension, not every one is religious. This suggests that spirituality and religion, although popularly seen as being similar if not the same are in fact different. Religion can be described as:

'...an organised system of beliefs, practices, rituals and symbols [that] facilitates closeness to the sacred or transcendent (God or higher power) [and which] fosters an understanding of man's relationship and responsibilities to others in living together in a community.'

MacKinlay (2006: 13)

Spirituality can be seen as:

'The personal quest for understanding answers to ultimate questions about life, about meaning and about relationships to the sacred or transcendent, which may [or may not] lead to or arise from the development of religious rituals and the formation of community.'

MacKinlay (2006: 13)

Spirituality could be seen as a solitary journey or quest undertaken by the individual without necessarily involving a recourse to a Deity (a Supreme Being, or a God) or to theological doctrine or formal religious teachings. Religion is very similar, although the same journey or quest may be undertaken as a community activity. Spirituality as a religion is an activity bound and given shape by rituals and rules, doctrines, teachings and resultant theology of a central figure. Religion is part of spirituality but not its totality, and spirituality is part of religion but not its totality.

Being a member of a religion, according to Stoter (1995), is being part of a particular cultural environment with particular beliefs, creeds and codes. The practice of religion is what, for many of us, gives spirituality a direction and purpose, as it helps (or should help) humans relate to the sacred. However, it must be remembered that performing a crude head count during a religious service does not equal religious participation: for example church attendance measures only church attendance and not the reason for attending. Neither does church attendance imply or signify religious or spiritual support wanted, given or received. However, it could be argued that many, if not most, of those who do attend places of worship are seeking support from a central figure, leaders of a faith, and from local faith communities and congregations. Boff (1985) suggests that encounters with a central figure is the core of religion and that people who seek ceremonies and rituals primarily may lose the purpose of religion which is to lead the individual person to the divine. However, it could be argued that a person who is drawn to ceremonies and rituals, for example one who is drawn to church music, may be starting out on a spiritual journey and experiencing the divine but on a sub-conscious level. It may, therefore, seem unfair and even inappropriate to believe that the person who is caught up and moved to tears by a beautiful painting or piece of music is not having as meaningful and even profound spiritual experience.

Spirituality and health care across the ages

In providing spiritual care or assisting service users to engage in their own spiritual journey there appears to be a focus on concentrating such delivery to service users who are elderly. However, would it be more accurate to say that any service user, regardless of age, would have spiritual needs that should be met?

The splitting of a person's life journey into discrete age sections can be found in many cultures. Each life stage is made distinguishable by specific ceremonies; each ceremony has its own associated spirituality. For example, within Western Christianity Christenings/baptism, Communion, Marriage, etc.

Within a non-religious context, similar age splits can be found. For example: the start of nursery school, leaving school, birth of own children, retirement, etc. Some of these life journeys have distinctive beginning and ending features, and in sociological literature these are described as 'rites of passage'.

According to MacKinlay (2006) the traditional Hindu views life as comprising four stages:

- Brahmacharya (childhood, from birth to marriage)
- Grihastha (begins at marriage)
- Vanaprastha (when your own children have reached adulthood)
- Sannyasa (old age, when the person renounces all worldly ties and spends all of their time in meditation and contemplation.

These four stages correspond roughly with the 'four ages' of man as proposed by MacKinlay (2006). Although the Hindu Sannyasa and the 'fourth age' of MacKinlay focuses on persons of very advanced years preparing for their end of life, it may be more accurate to say that this stage of the human's spiritual journey could occur at anytime from conception onwards. Thus, a more accurate way of looking at the 'fourth age' or Sannyasa is to view this stage as occurring concurrently with all other stages of human life. Therefore, it follows that it would be appropriate to assist a service user in an appropriate way at whatever stage of the spiritual journey they have reached. It would not be appropriate to assume that the person you are working with does not have spiritual needs simply because they are young, for example.

Practical considerations

First of all, spirituality does not lend itself to a 'tick chart' approach. Spiritual needs differ considerably from one person to another and expression and satisfaction of these needs are found in different ways (Stoter, 1995).

The healthcare assistant has a vital role in helping to assess and meet these needs. In order to meet these needs, the healthcare assistant must be aware of, understand and be comfortable with their own spirituality. Note, I am not suggesting that care staff need to be religious, as that is an entirely different issue. If care staff are not aware of their own spirituality or are comfortable with this it is debatable how and how far they can be comfortable with assisting another human being in a spiritually imposing way. It is very important not to impose your own beliefs on another person. Seeking an understanding of the self as a spiritual being will not be easy: where does one start? There are large numbers of easily obtainable popular magazines and self-help books on the subject, most of which tend to promote, and be seen as part of popular lifestyles, and this also includes lifestyle TV programmes. The problem with these is that they tend to lack any real depth, dealing with spirituality at a very superficial level.

One of the fundamental duties of a healthcare assistant is the assessment of what a patient or a service user wishes to access in terms of the meeting of religious or spiritual needs. Individuals who have strong beliefs or who follow a particular religion will let you know of this when you are asking routine admission questions on this. Others, including the patient or service user's close relatives or friends will indicate they wish to talk to someone about this as a particular event unfolds. Although it is a key principle that helping a patient or service user meet spiritual needs is not amenable to a tick-box assessment exercise, there are nonetheless a number of such assessment tools and your employing organisation might use one of these. MacKinlay (2006) designed an assessment tool mainly for use with older people. However, the drawback with some tools is that they are designed to be used specifically with elderly people. However, with some creative and imaginative thought this assessment tool could be modified and adapted for use across all ages, abilities/disabilities, health and social care conditions and work settings. Any resultant care plans will necessitate liaising and working across many professional boundaries.

Healthcare assistants must recognise that participation in a religion and its practices is for many people a very important aspect of their lives. This recognition should lead to assisting those service users who express a need to access places of worship or at the very least a minister of their chosen religion. Whilst you might not share such religious beliefs, you have a duty to recognise that a patient or a service user has clearly stated or recognisable religious needs that require to be met. You must act on this recognition otherwise you are denying the patient or service user a dignity and respect which is theirs by right. It is not appropriate here to have a 'one size fits all' approach to religious participation. By this is meant that it is not appropriate to treat Christians, Jews, Muslims, and Hindus, for example, alike and procure the services of the local Anglican vicar to provide religious and spiritual help. It is even inappropriate to treat all Christians, for example, as being the same and having the same needs, as there are theological and doctrinal differences within Christianity. Such engagement may involve asking the appropriate religious leader or clergy to visit the patient, being aware of religious festivals and cultural needs such as diet and care provision, or taking the patient or service user, if possible, to their preferred place of worship (this is likely to be more possible if you work in a residential or nursing home and there is enough staff available to facilitate this).

Another important role that you have as a healthcare assistant is how you act when you are around the patient or service user — do you come across as being hurried with little time for a smile and a chat? Are you always hurried or, despite being busy, do you present a sense of stillness and even peace? Are you at peace with yourself, others and the environment? How cluttered is your working environment? These may seem to be somewhat odd questions to ask within today's health and social care world of busyness, targets, cutbacks, service reconfigurations and stress. However, if you are to accompany your service user, resident, or patient in their spiritual journey at possibly some of the most vulnerable and yet challenging times in their lives, how can you do so if you are always in a state of physical and spiritual clutter, unrest and turmoil? Even during a hectic work day with many calls on your time and attention it is vital that you remember that the person with whom you are working is a human being first and foremost and not a physical or mental health condition. Relate to them as a human on a human level with a sense of genuine care, attention and stillness. Let them realize that they are the most important person in your life at that specific moment. Even the most seemingly mundane of tasks, such as assisting a person to use the toilet, to have a wash, to dry themselves, to get dressed or undressed or to eat, if undertaken in an attitude of humility, care and love can be transformed into a spiritual moment for the patient, service user or resident, and for you as the care giver.

Conclusion

Spirituality within the context of health and social care was never going to be an easy subject to cover in such short a space as this, and I hope that I have done it justice. I also hope that this short chapter on spirituality has been of interest and help to you in your daily work and your engagement with your patient's or service user's spiritual journey and, indeed, in your own spiritual journey. Remember that spirituality is not about filling in a tick-box assessment, nor is it an optional extra. Meeting a person's spiritual need is a vital component of care, irrespective of the setting or the context of care delivery. The role of any healthcare professional is to provide a holistic care, and therefore due consideration to the spiritual needs of patients and service users is not something to be ignored or from which we can opt out.

Boff L (1985) *Church: charism and power.* SCM Press Ltd, London

MacKinlay E (2006) *Spiritual growth and care in the fourth age of life.* Jessica Kingsley Publishers, London

McSherry W (2007) *The meaning of spirituality and spiritual care within nursing and health care practice.* Quay Books, London

Stoter D (1995) *Spiritual aspects of health care.* Mosby, London

CHAPTER 15

Work-based learning

Angela Grainger

The aim of this chapter is to help you to maximise the various type of learning opportunities that exist in the workplace; the work place also constituting the patient care environment. It is generally well accepted that personal satisfaction often comes from a sense of having made the best decisions, and that staff usually want to do perform well at work and to enjoy their job (Evans, 1985).

Why learning is important

Positive feedback from our patients and from our managers helps to improve our self esteem because our work has been recognised as making a significant contribution to patient care. It is affirmed in our mind that we have performed well and that this is appreciated, so consequently we wish to repeat this experience.

It is important to remember that constructive criticism given properly helps us to understand what we could have done better or differently and to take this into account when approaching the next similar situation. Remembering that we are in a privileged position to attend to our patients' needs and that the patients are the central focus of all that we do helps us to accept that sometimes we need to receive constructive criticism as well as praise. Moreover, the benefit that follows from listening to constructive criticism and gaining understanding as to why we need to do something differently is seen in the improvements made to patient care, which cyclically brings us back to the starting point that healthcare staff are motivated to want to give good care and to do well at work.

A person's attitude is also closely associated with the ability to acquire new and further knowledge. Motivation is the key to learning because if we want to know something we are likely to learn it. Self knowledge is at the heart of individual development (Evans, 1985). Remember, too, that yesterday's junior members of the healthcare team tend to be the senior leaders of tomorrow therefore 'learning on the job' in order to perfect our performance is a necessary part of growing up in the job and acquiring the required competences for not only the job in hand but also for gaining promotional opportunities.

Defining work-based learning

Work-based learning can be defined as the influences in the workplace that shape a member of staff's behaviour and attitude through exposure to activities and experiences which promote knowledge and enhance skills so that a competent work performance is achieved.

Adults learn from experience. As an adult learner you will know how you come to make sense of things, and how you remember, recall, and apply them. How effective learning occurs and the factors that facilitate this is the remit of educationalists and educational psychologists.

In the following sections I give a brief explanation as to how learning, and in particular experiential learning, help enhance learning abilities.

Experiential learning and how this works

Kolb (1976) has helped us understand how learning is acquired from experience. New actions constitute new experiences, which begin a new cycle of learning. By building on the initial skills or competences achieved we are developing a further capacity to learn more, and therefore to be able to do more. Experience can lead to significant learning so that not all learning has to take place in a formally structured way in a classroom. For Kolb (1976) an actual lived experience — known as a *concrete experience* because something tangible has been encountered — leads to reflective observation as to what happened and why, what worked well and what did not. This in turn leads to abstract conceptualisation whereby the learner seeks the knowledge (the theoretical understanding) that can be applied to the same or a similar future situation in order to ensure a better outcome. Finally, the learner is thinking on his/her feet and is applying the knowledge and skills gained from the previous stages (concrete experience, reflective observation, and abstract conceptualisation) to the situation facing him/her and undertakes relevant active experimentation to try and improve matters.

A practical example would be the concrete experience a healtcare assistant is having in facing a patient who is unhappy with the nursing care and who has a distrustful relative. Reflective observation occurs when the healthcare assistant asks the registered nurse to speak to the patient and to the relative and observes what the registered nurse does to try and find out the underlying cause of the unhappiness and the measures taken to put the patient and the relative at their ease and to improve the situation. Abstract conceptualisation occurs when the healthcare assistant asks the registered nurse why he/she responded to the patient and to the relative in a certain way, and what actions were taken and why, in order to gain a further understanding of the whole situation. Later, the healthcare assistant might read an article on how to allay the fears and anxieties of patients and relatives, and perhaps another article on handling patients' complaints so that a factual understanding of accepted good practice, known as evidence-based practice, is obtained. This additional factual knowledge is likely to be stored in that part of the brain dealing with the memory and recalled when a similar future situation is encountered.

The active experimentation phase of learning is actually an appropriative creative response to a situation. In the above-mentioned scenario the healthcare assistant will interpret the verbal and non-verbal body language cues of the patient and the relative as indicating they are dissatisfied or concerned about something. The healthcare assistant then initiates action by politely enquiring if anything is the matter and can he/she do anything to help. Providing the patient is not nil-by-mouth, a cup of tea might help the patient and or the relative to unwind a little and to tell the healthcare assistant what is troubling them. Whilst the healthcare assistant will still inform the registered nurse who will come and see the patient and the relative, the healthcare assistant has done a lot to ensure that the registered nurse is not walking into a situation without some very good background preparation. The healthcare assistant has therefore more than adequately fulfilled his/her role in being of assistance to the patient and to the relative, and to the registered nurse.

Healthcare staff need to acquire competences that require learning in the cognitive and the affective domains. What this means is that the theory applied to the practicalities of care is learned by thinking about this in order that the theory relates to the required associated knowledge, i.e. the 'knowing' (cognition). The values and attitudes that influence how care is delivered and therefore experienced by the patient is learned by engaging the affective domain of the learner's brain. Being at work and coming into contact with all sorts of patients who are facing all sorts of situations allows us to learn from our patients. We also meet colleagues who are members of the multidisciplinary team and who therefore complement the care we, as members of the nursing family, give to patients so that the patients total needs are met. Like ourselves and our colleagues, patients are from different cultural backgrounds so we get to mix with many interesting people from all walks of life. When you take these factors into account, and the fact that our employing organisations also regularly undergo changes in order to meet the changing needs of society, we can see that we are in a prime position at work to maximise learning opportunities.

Making use of all our senses when learning

In the table below (*Table 1*) Quinn (2000) an explanation is given for the following learning terms and for how learning is assessed.

It is important to remember that once we become competent in performing a skill that we are required to perform several times in succession, such as a blanket bath or emptying a catheter bag, we run the risk of becoming 'habitual performers' because what we are doing is so routine to us. Although the giving of technical competent care is important it is not the whole story. Patients also require technically competent care to be given with compassion and for their individual needs to be met. Neither healthcare professionals nor their patients are automatons so the human experience of being with each other and in having socially and therapeutically sensitive interactions is vital to the work we do.

Types of work-based or self directed learning opportunities

How can you become aware of the various learning opportunities available to us?

Know your job description
Be familiar with your job description as this explains in general terms what role you are being employed to do and therefore the duties you are expected to undertake and need to become proficient at. Some competences are related to the pay/salary scale for the grade/banding of the post.

Local induction
If you are new in post then you should have a local induction. The purpose of an induction period is to allow you to become familiar with your working environment, to get to know your colleagues, and to know important health and safety procedures such as fire evacuation, and also any policies and procedures your employer requires you to follow such as reporting sick, and booking annual leave, etc. You may also be required to attend a corporate induction which explains the employing organisation's values and the way in which it conducts its work.

Clinical supervision/mentoring
A healthcare assistant who has an accredited qualification such as a National Vocational Qualification or Scottish Vocational Qualification (NVQ/SVQ)

Table 1. Learning terms and how learning is assessed

The cognitive (thinking) domain		
Knowledge	Possessing key, relevant facts	Identifies, names, states
Comprehension	Understanding	Explains, gives examples
Application	Applies rules and principles and understanding to real situations	Demonstrates, uses, prepares and produces
Analysis	Breaks down information into component parts from the less important to the most important	Differentiates and distinguishes
Synthesis	Combines the various parts of learning into a whole product of knowledge and understanding	Composes a plan, for example a care plan
Evaluation	The ability to make judgements and therefore prioritise thoughts and actions	Justifies, compares and contrasts
The affective (feeling domain)		
Receiving	Actively listens	Pays attention, responds appropriately to questions
Responds	Actively engages	Responds to and follows instructions
Valuing	Joining in	Participates in discussion and other activities, has a degree of empathy and understands how the patient is feeling

Organisation	Arranges work (care-giving) in a relevant and logical pattern, performs duties smoothly	Good time-keeping, aware of own competence an seeks help when required
The psychomotor domain		
Perception	Responds to sensory cues	Awareness of non-verbal body language and interprets this accurately
Guided response	Practices following a demonstration	Engages in learning by watching and asking relevant questions
Mechanical performance	Repeated practice of a set skill	Manual dexterity giving a gentle and deft (skilled) performance, consistent good performance each time

Source: Adapted Quinn (2000)

Level 3 might be assigned to you as a clinical supervisor and work-helpmate. Do not be in awe of this arrangement. Remember we all started at the beginning and worked our way up to senior positions. You will be the one acting as the helpmate/buddy in the future. This is about accessing and taking advantage of competent companionship.

Establishing a relationship with your clinical supervisor/work buddy
Discuss with your supervisor/work-helpmate/buddy how the arrangement is supposed to work. When the ice has been broken and you have got to know each other, do try and talk about anything that you might have a concern about early on because the longer you leave this, the harder it can get to initiate this type of conversation.

Tapping into your employer's education lead
Large employing organisations tend to have education managers in post, if this is not the case one of the senior managers will oversee this function. Please remember that your line manager shares a joint responsibility with you to enhance your access to relevant learning opportunities — after all your manager wants you to do a good job too. If you feel you have a problem with basic literacy or basic numerical skills and that this might affect your

ability to write care plans or to measure and chart fluids, then please do raise this with either your supervisor/work buddy or your line manager as help can be obtained. If you really feel you cannot talk directly them about this then if you are a union member you can contact either the local steward or the local learning representative who can help you.

Using competence assessment documents

If your employer gives you a competence assessment document or you are undertaking work-based learning for an accredited vocational qualification and have a competence assessment document for this, then ensure you have this with you every time you are on duty and that you keep this in a presentable form. This document is a record of your achievements and should be completed every time a new competence is acquired, which your supervisor then signs off as having been achieved.

Accepting constructive criticism

Be prepared to accept constructive criticism (that which is given for a clearly justifiable reason, delivered calmly and politely in a private place) with good grace. Take note of what is said and why and be prepared to alter any similar future care-giving so that it is performed in the correct manner as previously explained.

Journal clubs

Read relevant articles in healthcare journals. Your organisation might have a journal club where staff meet to discuss the content of a relevant article and healthcare assistants usually join in with this or have a similar event for themselves where issues relevant to the healthcare assistant role are discussed.

Conferences

Try to attend a conference designed to meet the needs of the healthcare assistant. Several organisations and unions/staff professional associations are now hosting these. If you cannot attend then read about the conference content in one of the healthcare journals.

E-learning programmes

Many large organisations now have their own, or have purchased, e-learning programmes, which are relatively easy to use via the internet. Some have a multiple choice format so that if you give the correct answer you can then move on to the next question. Completion of the programme often allows you to print off a certificate of completion which you could then add to your portfolio of learning.

Mandatory training

Attend all mandatory in-house training such as moving and handling training and the legally required update training. Other examples of in-house training include infection control and good hygiene practice, food handling hygiene standards, and basic life support. You might also be taught how to use a computerised electronic recording system for tracking and obtaining patients' records and for documenting care-giving.

Learning logs — part of a portfolio of development

Maintain a learning log which reflects back anything that you feel has led you to acquire further and deeper significant learning. Examples might include dealing with very distressed relatives, involvement in a cardiac arrest situation, or physically assisting a patient to eat and drink whose involuntary bodily movements made this particularly problematic. It might even reflect how you dealt with the situation where for the first time you are the buddy/workmate and demonstrated how a skill should be performed to a new healthcare assistant.

I have found that a good tip for starting a learning log is to purchase a hard-backed blank journal that has a cover design which you like. This personalises it and makes you feel you want to write in it. Do not feel you have to record something every day as this can make what is meant to be a pleasurable activity feel tedious. Record events that have happened that are of significance to you and remember to capture not only what happened and what you did but also what you felt about the event. Maintain confidentiality by making anonymous the real identities of the actual people involved. Refer to patients as 'patient X and to colleagues as 'healthcare assistant Y' or 'staff nurse P', etc.

If you have not recorded anything in your learning log for about three months or more then take a few minutes to think back about generally what has happened at work and how you feel, and record this. I have found that I can look back in my learning logs and identify the significant skills I learned at a particular stage in time. This has proved very useful when asked at interview a question such as: *'What's the most difficult thing you have had to handle and what did you learn from this?'* because you can speak from reality and therefore give a more credible response.

Linking work-based learning with more formal learning

Talk to your organisation's education lead, to your manager, or to your clinical supervisor about the possibility of undertaking an NVQ/SVQ or equivalent qualification. Check out the website for this and the website for Skills for Life/Skills for Health. The Open University also offers modular study relevant to healthcare assistants and their work. Some healthcare assistants will wish to undertake statutory nurse training in order to become a registered nurse or midwife. If so, please talk to your line manager or your employer's education lead about this as some organisations will second healthcare assistants for this. It is also a good idea to look at the websites and the prospectuses of the various universities offering statutory nursing and midwifery training.

Investing in your career; the role of appraisals and of personal development plans

By taking advantage of all the various learning opportunities available you are investing in your self and your career. Super (1980) describes this type of investment as a 'career rainbow' because it runs alongside all the learning you have acquired as part of the various life stages you have gone through such as being a child, a student, a partner, a parent, and being, or preparing to be, an older person.

During the course of your employment you will also probably have an annual appraisal with your line manager. The purpose of the appraisal is for you and your line manager to jointly look at your progress during the year against the required competences set out in your job description. This is not a punitive (punishing) exercise. The appraisal is so that you receive your line manager's recognition for the contribution you have made to the service, and for the progress you have made in acquiring new competences, and in perfecting to a high-art form those that you were previously performing at a novice or a beginner's stage.

A *personal development plan* is where at the end of the appraisal you agree with your manager your next continuing professional development. This is a plan of action designed to meet set goals or objectives, so do not be afraid to inform your line manager as to what you wish to do in the short and longer-term as it is only with this knowledge that we can help to assist you in achieving your dream.

Benner (1984) explains how all of us start by beginning to learn a competence as a relatively unknowing novice, and that by practising under competent guidance we become an advanced beginner. By continuously practising our craft and by taking advantage of further learning opportunities we become competent and can often be left to perform a skill, or a distinctive aspect of work, on our own. The highest level of achievement is that of expert practitioner which is where the level of knowledge, understanding and competence is so high that the healthcare professional is proactive in identifying subtle changes in the patient's condition and therefore takes appropriate action to minimise the risk of complications occurring.

Competence is not just achieved by watching and then doing. It requires us to think about what we are doing and to seek feedback as to how we are doing from a reliable, knowledgeable and credible source. This can be feedback from, for example, your clinical supervisor/work buddy, from the content of an article in a healthcare journal, and from the answer responses you get from engaging in an interactive e-learning programme. You can also get feedback on a more personal and intimate level by undertaking reflective practice.

Reflective practice

Reflection is where you think back on something that has occurred and focus on putting the events in sequential order, identifying the causative factors that led to or contributed to the event. The purpose of reflective practice is to think about what went wrong or what went well and to identify what would be better practice should we face this situation again. It is a form of self-directed learning for those who have a conscience and a motivation to do the very best that they can. You therefore have to be personally honest about your own feelings and whether this might have influenced the turn of events.

For example, a patient is reluctant to have a bath at the time that would be convenient to the staff, given everything else that is going on in the care area at that particular time. You are new to the workplace and want to make a good impression. You know that the registered nurse wishes the patient to have the bath, and this particular nursing duty has been assigned to you. You get on well with the patient and you are able to persuade the patient, without any form of coercion, to have the bath. You naturally feel pleased about this. Later you find that the patient is refusing to have lunch and is tearful.

Reflective practice helps us to put everything into the picture and to gain a perspective of what really happened, rather than what we would like to think has happened. Reflective practice can be done individually, in a one-one situation with a clinical supervisor, or in small groups depending on what it is that is being reflected on. In the example above, individual reflection and/or one-to-one reflection would be appropriate.

Group reflection would be appropriate when a situation involves or affects a number of staff. For example, a much loved patient suddenly and unexpectedly dies and the relatives, after a reasonable time has elapsed, continue to be difficult and demanding. Further insightful knowledge and greater competence often results from reflective practice.

As Bolton (2001) explains, reflection is a panoramic view of the complete scenario, and includes taking account of the views of others, whilst reflexivity pays attention to one's own actions, thoughts and feelings and how these have interacted to shape the overall event.

Reflection is often after an event, but very experienced practitioners are able to 'reflect in practice' meaning that they reflect as things are happening and as a situation is unfolding in order to take action that avoids the situation getting any worse. Being honest with ourselves in recalling what we did and how we now feel about that requires a degree of emotional maturity.

Emotional intelligence and the management of stress

The work of Goleman (1995) has highlighted that people respond to situations and circumstances not so much from having logical rational thought processes, but rather from associated emotional feelings that accompany the picture they see. This is perfectly normal but on occasions can get out of hand and be a cause of stress. For example, a healthcare worker who was overly criticised as a child might fear failure and therefore be reluctant to engage in learning opportunities. Moreover, instead of being able to accept constructive criticism with good grace, and to move on from this, the healthcare worker might respond by denying anything is wrong and instead be overly critical of colleagues.

The reason we need to acquire an emotionally intelligent response to situations is so that we can continue to learn and to grow, and very importantly to manage our stress levels. Life is stressful and healthcare work is stressful, so it is important that you identify what are your personal stressors and how you manage these.

Taking your allotted break times and managing your time properly eases stress build-up. This calls for team-working so that the workload does not become the burden of just one or two people. Very often conscientious staff find themselves naturally taking on more and more work. It is important to know when to say: '*No, I cannot work in this way anymore*', and to discuss this with your line manager.

Managing other life stressors along with work needs some thought and pre-planning. Moving house might be better during an annual leave period rather than trying to work all day and sorting a new house out in the evening. Work-home life or personal space balance is important. The old saying of all work and no play makes for a dull person is very apt. Understanding and managing the frustrations of others who closely interact with you is key to not feeling pulled in all directions. Sometimes family and friends can feel you are neglecting them in favour of giving care to a lot of strangers, even though this is your work. Negotiate times for when you can be with them.

Proper assertiveness, which is distinguishable from aggression, is a core skill for most healthcare professionals, and many organisations offer this training as part of a communications skills package. Reflecting on the strength of any feelings you might have in relation to a particular situation or incident can help you acquire insight into why these feelings might be so strong. Strong feelings are perfectly alright but it is reassuring to know for ourselves where these come from; it is when strong feelings become overwhelming that leads to the problem of stress. The stress can affect just the individual concerned on a personal level but if this spills over into the work situation and is of such magnitude it can also affect the team working with that individual. We therefore owe it to ourselves and to each other to know what 'makes us tick' and to think about whether how we react to things either upsets or causes irritation to others.

Do remember though that you are allowed to be human. We are still growing up in certain situations, mainly those that we have not encountered before, for example, such as our experiencing the death of our own loved ones. We do not know how we would cope with grieving and bereavement until it happens to us. My advice is to get to know yourself well, be your own best friend and look after yourself. Investing in all relevant learning opportunities is a very good habit that will help you with this.

Conclusion

This chapter has explained the meaning of work-based learning and has discussed the various practical ways in which you can maximise work-based learning opportunities so that you can continue ti build-up knowledge and competence in order that patient care is of a high quality. Working in healthcare is very rewarding, but on occasions it can also be demanding and stressful and this chapter has additionally looked at how you can undertake some self-directed learning on stress management. This chapter has also explored the meaning of emotional intelligence and how gaining this can improve our responses to stressful situations, which might include that of unblocking and to help us improve our overall work performance so that we can progress to achieving further and more advances competences, which in turn enhances our feeling of job satisfaction.

Bolton G (2001) *Reflective Practice, Writing and Professional Development*. Paul Chapman Publishing Limited, London

Benner P (1984) *From Novice to Expert. Excellence and Power in Clinical Nursing Practice*. Addison Wesley, Menlo-Park

Evans N (1985) *Post-Education Society: Recognising Adults as Learners*. Croom Helm Ltd, Kent

Goleman D (1995) *Emotional Intelligence.* Guildford Press, New York

Kolby D (1976) *Learning Style Inventory.* McBer and Company, Boston

Quinn FM (2000) *The Principles and Practice of Nurse Education.* Stanley Thornes, London

Super D (1980) A lifespan, life space approach to career development. *Journal of Vocational Behaviour* **16:** 46

INDEX